"In a time when labels are meaningless, Sacks cuts through consumer confusion and tells the truth about our food system. *What the Fork Are You Eating?* is an informative, accessible guide on how to choose healthy—and safe—food. A must-read for anyone who cares about what they put in their body."

—**ANTHONY FASSIO**, CEO, Natural Gourmet Institute

"Stefanie reminds us to *slow the fork down*, encouraging us to learn the story behind our food so that we can make better food choices that will truly nourish our body, mind, and spirit." —**RICHARD MCCARTHY**, executive director, Slow Food USA®

"In a world where our children are expected to have shorter life spans than ourselves and where the leading cause of death for children under fifteen is cancer, it is imperative that we are all educated on our food choices. *What the Fork Are You Eating?* is an invaluable tool to help you feed yourself, your family, and your friends the 'best,' healthiest food possible. With Stefanie Sacks as your guide, you can positively impact the health of your family, our food supply, and possibly our planet as well!"

—**ANN COOPER**, founder of the Chef Ann Foundation and author of *Lunch Lessons: Changing the Way We Feed Our Children*

"Stefanie Sacks really stirs the pot in her must-read book, *What the Fork Are You Eating?* With wit, wisdom, and authority, Stefanie clearly lays out what nasty additives are hiding in our food, and empowers us with concrete solutions on how to make cleaner food choices. This book is a must-have for all of us looking to enhance our health and well-being."

—**REBECCA KATZ**, MS, author of *The Cancer-Fighting Kitchen* and *The Longevity Kitchen*

"There's a revolution coming, and the most powerful weapon is your fork! You choose—is your fork a weapon of mass destruction, or does it wield food as medicine? In *What the Fork Are You Eating?* Stefanie Sacks tells you what the fork to do to ward off the Top-Rated Terminators, and get yourself to pantry and meal rehab for a longer and healthier life!"

—**MARY BETH AUGUSTINE**, MS, RDN, CDN, director of nutrition, Saybrook University, and author of *The Detox Prescription*

"Stefanie Sacks asks the pressing question, 'When will the food industry and the government stop playing roulette with our health?' She elucidates myriad ways they are doing so, as well as how we can navigate a healthy route through our food system. This book is an invaluable resource in guiding each one of us to be part of the solution."

—MARY CLEAVER, chef and owner of The Cleaver Company and The Green Table

"Stefanie Sacks has given us an eminently practical guide to help us navigate the windy road of healthy eating. Her expertise in this field is evident on every page as she lays out in straightforward language the dangers of the artificial food industry and the Better for You Alternatives. Her good-natured approach is a refreshing change from the fear-based messages we find so often in books about nutrition. As a pediatrician, I will be recommending this book to all my families to support mindful, healthy eating. Enjoy each chapter of *What the Fork* as you would a good meal. Bon appetit."

—STEPHEN COWAN, MD, FAAP, author of *Fire Child, Water Child: How Understanding the Five Types of ADHD Can Help You Improve Your Child's Self-Esteem and Attention*

WHAT THE FORK
Are You Eating?

WHAT THE FORK
Are You Eating?

An Action Plan for Your Pantry and Plate

Stefanie Sacks, MS, CNS, CDN

JEREMY P. TARCHER • PENGUIN
a member of Penguin Group (USA)
New York

JEREMY P. TARCHER/PENGUIN
Published by the Penguin Group
Penguin Group (USA) LLC
375 Hudson Street
New York, New York 10014

USA · Canada · UK · Ireland · Australia
New Zealand · India · South Africa · China

penguin.com
A Penguin Random House Company

Most Tarcher/Penguin books are available at special quantity discounts for bulk purchase for sales promotions,
premiums, fund-raising, and educational needs. Special books or book excerpts also can be created to fit
specific needs. For details, write: Special.Markets@us.penguingroup.com.

Library of Congress Cataloging-in-Publication Data

Sacks, Stefanie.
What the fork are you eating? : an action plan for your pantry and plate / Stefanie Sacks, MS, CNS, CDN.
p.   cm.
Includes bibliographical references and index.
ISBN 978-0-399-16796-6
1. Natural foods.   2. Grocery shopping.   3. Food additives.   4. Nutrition.   I. Title.
TX369.S23   2014   2014027015
641.3'02—dc23

Printed in the United States of America
1   3   5   7   9   10   8   6   4   2

Book design by Gretchen Achilles

Life begins at the end of your comfort zone.

—NEALE DONALD WALSCH

Contents

Foreword

My dear friend and nutritional sounding board Stefanie Sacks is an impassioned food warrior—just listen to her wonderful public radio show, WPPB's *Stirring the Pot*. She represents the yin and yang of healthy food advocacy—the love of delicious, nourishing food and the zeal for holding the food industry's feet to the fire, blowing the whistle on the cheap sugar, fat, salt, and weird industrial chemicals getting poured into processed foods that dominate the supermarket. Now you, the reader, can make your voice heard with your fork.

I first met Stefanie almost twenty years ago when I was the director of nutrition at the Canyon Ranch spa in the Berkshires in western Massachusetts. She had recently graduated from culinary school and was beginning her master's degree in nutrition education at Teachers College, Columbia University. She sought me out, eager even then, because she recognized that we shared a common passion—we were both nutritionists (or, in her case, a budding nutritionist) who loved food and cooking. Back then, that combination wasn't so easy to find!

Fast forward ten years, and I'm at the prestigious Integrative Healthcare Symposium in Manhattan listening to a presentation given by Stefanie and another cutting-edge nutritionist friend of mine, Mary Beth Augustine, MS, RDN, CDN. They emphasized the harms that the food component gluten, found in many grains and in so much of our food supply, could do to digestion and to overall health. This was before gluten had become a trendy nutritional hot-button issue. As someone who had once suffered from an undiagnosed sensitivity to gluten, I was impressed with their marshaling of the scientific evidence and the conviction they brought to their presentation. When Stefanie and I compared notes later on, we weren't surprised to find that we'd both struggled with chronic unwellness in our earlier years. Like a lot of the most committed people in our field, we'd been to hell with our own health and we had found our way out by changing our diet. It's that story that drives her passion to share what she knows with her clients and now her readers. It's what steels her backbone to challenge the nutritional status quo.

I discovered Stefanie's love of food and the joy she takes in being in the kitchen over these past five years leading nutrition and culinary workshops with her at the Kripalu Center for Yoga and Health, one of the landmark wellness centers in the Berkshires. She also brings her knowledge and culinary toolkit to the national educational course I organize every year for the Center for Mind-Body Medicine called "Food As Medicine." Stefanie, one of my "cooks on call," leads food demos and shares insights with the conference faculty and participants.

A course taught by Stefanie is like no other. In one, we blindfolded the students to put them in closer touch with the sensory experience of food. In just about all of our shared workshops, she cranked up the music, and when we weren't cooking, we were dancing. She was probably the most "tuned-in" person I've ever shared a kitchen with. Everything was beautifully organized. And she met each student where they were at, going over basic knife skills with the beginners so they could safely shed their fears and trading treasured recipes with the advanced students, some of whom had worked in professional kitchens.

In *What the Fork Are You Eating?* Stefanie has taken on a serious and daunting project—getting rid of the bad food in our diet and replacing it with what's better—and made it manageable for a wide range of readers, neophytes and the nutritional mavens alike. In researching and writing this book, she's become a formidable expert on the issues, one on whom I rely for the latest and best information (I brought *The Swift Diet: 4 Weeks to Mend the Belly, Lose the Weight, and Get Rid of the Bloat* into this world at about the same time Stefanie was working on this book; our regular check-in phone calls were to me, and I hope to her, an invaluable resource).

But for all the knowledge she's amassed, her approach is refreshingly practical—an "action plan," she calls it. Her goal isn't organic purity; *it's getting rid of the crap.* This book reminds me of the courses we teach. There and here, Stefanie wields a sharp knife, zealously, and with love.

—KATHIE MADONNA SWIFT, MS, RDN, LDN

Introduction

Having immersed myself in the world of food, nutrition, and health since the ripe age of fifteen, I have been there, done that—raw, vegan, vegetarian, macrobiotic, special medical diets including cleanses, and yes (I am ashamed to say so), even fad diets. Let's call it my years of necessary research. As a result, I am proud that I have become a true *moderationist*—I don't follow any one food theory or fad, I don't eat 100 percent organic, I eat some packaged foods and I eat not-so-healthy foods once in a while (a good potato chip is my vice, even the occasional gummy bear—more on this later). But at the same time, I practice no-nonsense nutrition—meaning I don't buy into any of the hype; I believe in real food, not phony food (as in highly processed food); and I tell it like it is, always coming from a place of facts and basic logic.

Suffering from asthma, allergies, recurring bronchitis, and pneumonia shaped much of my childhood, and I was determined to find an alternative to the multiple inhalers, allergy meds, steroids, and antibiotics I regularly consumed. In a nutshell, the medications that were supposed to be helping me were actually destroying me. Based on my experience as a summer chef in my local Montauk health food café, I discovered ways I could use food to help me heal. Challenged to the core, but finally getting well, I learned two things that shaped my life as I now know it:

- I truly understood the power that food has to influence a body's ability to heal, recover from chronic illness, and stay well.
- I began questioning why more people didn't know about this, and even if they did, I wondered whether they would have the knowledge and skills to make the shift that I did.

As I figured out how to turn my food passion and fascination into a career, I also discovered my mission: to teach what I'd learned in my idiosyncratic no-nonsense nutritionist way.

I am a culinary nutritionist—a certified chef with a master's of science degree in nutrition from Columbia University. I am also a certified nutrition specialist (CNS) and a certified dietitian nutritionist (CDN). Many clients call me a food therapist. A doctor who suggests dietary change as a part of the prescription for healing typically hands over a single sheet offering minimal guidance. I work with clients to take this "nutrition prescription" into the kitchen—we chat, shop, and cook, as I aim to do with you in this book.

What the Fork is a digestible read. You may move through it quickly or take it in stages. Either way, hopefully you will benefit from the information and tools offered. Learn about the things in your food or being done to your food that are just not cool with the Top-Rated Terminators, including what they are, why they are "bad," and how to avoid them with the Better for You Alternatives (to whet your appetite for your trip to the market in Section Three). Then let's feng shui your food with Pantry Rehab before I help you navigate the grocery store, from decoding Nutrition Facts, ingredient lists, health claims, and funny (and not-so-funny) food lingo to aisle-by-aisle actionables in Supermarket Strategies. And last but not least, learn to love what you eat in Meal Rehab—you'll get tips on how to balance your plate as well as recipes to die for.

I am not a doctor or dietitian drilling down on a weight-loss solution; I am not offering a polemic on a food system gone awry (though you will get some serious insight on that here). Rather my intention is to give you enough information to push you to question *What the Fork* you are eating while also giving you the tools to start to do something about it. Never forget that small changes in food choice can make big everyday differences. I promote a more conscious way of choosing food—what could be bad about that?

Top-Rated Terminators

Before taking a close look at what the fork you are eating, a little background on how the federal government regulates food is necessary. Perhaps this will shed a little light on why many of the Top-Rated Terminators are in your edibles in the first place.

The 411 on Food Regulations

Today, your food is regulated through the joint efforts of several agencies. In a nutshell, the U.S. Department of Agriculture (USDA) keeps an eye on all the plants that are grown and animals raised in their natural habitat, while the Food and Drug Administration (FDA) ensures that your products (and drugs) are safe for consumption. As there are many harmful chemicals added to food, the Environmental Protection Agency (EPA) also gets involved to ensure that these substances remain at subtoxic levels so everything you ingest is positively protected.

It all started in 1862 when Abraham Lincoln established the USDA, marking the beginning of some level of food regulation. Then in the early 1900s, as more products began to hit the market, so did many untested chemicals in food. These included borax (a mineral and salt that has a mild toxicity level) and formaldehyde (a gaseous compound of high toxicity), both of which were added for preservation without consideration or knowledge of potential health consequences. Thanks to Dr. Harvey Wiley, chief chemist of the USDA's Bureau of Chemistry, Congress allocated funds to start testing the true safety of food products (with the scientific tools that existed at the time).

In 1906 the Pure Food and Drug Act was passed. It prohibited misbranded or adulterated foods, drinks, and drugs as well as the addition of color that masked inferiority in foods and even some colors that were poisonous. The concept was great but there was one major problem: There was no mandatory premarket testing of foods, so how could the government ensure true safety? Food was still a free-for-all.

But in 1914, after several amendments to the Pure Food and Drug Act (including regulations on what colors were safe as additives and how to label foods), the government finally decided that it was critical to show the effect that a chemical additive had on humans. Now the industry had to be accountable for the compounds they were slipping into your food.

However, even with these directives in place, food companies did their darnedest to dupe the consumer with chemicals and inferior ingredients. Take Bred Spred—an imitation jam introduced in the 1920s. According to FDA historian Suzanne White Junod, PhD, "There wasn't a single strawberry in the jar. It was made of coal tar, artificial pectin, artificial flavors, and grass seeds."[1]

Yet Americans didn't really care, as they didn't know any better—Bred Spred was packaged to perfection and *cost less* than the real deal. The 1920s marked the beginning of an era when packaged goods like Bred Spred gained supermarket shelf space.

In 1933 the Food and Drug Administration was birthed out of the USDA's Bureau of Chemistry, and in 1938 the Food, Drug, and Cosmetic Act (FD&C Act) was introduced to protect the consumer from deceptive foods. However, it seemed that unsavory substances were still getting into edibles, prompting the 1958 Food Additives Amendment, whereby manufacturers of new food additives had to establish said ingredients' safety to the satisfaction of the FDA before use.

Just so you are clear, according to the FDA, a food additive is a substance that has *no proven track record of safety* and must therefore undergo testing for approval by the FDA *before* it can be used in a food. However, there are plenty of ingredients in the foods you eat every day that are not defined as *additives* by the FDA, but as *generally recognized as safe (GRAS)* because they have been:

1. deemed "safe" by FDA scientists for intended use based on "published studies, which may be corroborated by unpublished studies and other data and information" and
2. used in food for a long period of time (with no "scientifically based" concerns); thus their use is exempt from FDA approval.[2]

On those studies that support the FDA in deeming a foodstuff safe (see item 1 above)—in 1973 the FDA granted propylene glycol (PG) GRAS status for its use in foods such as confections and frostings, frozen dairy products, seasonings, nuts, and nut products to keep the moisture in. It can also be found in nonfood items including cosmetics, detergents, paints, and coatings. While PG appears to be safe at low levels, it is important to note that in 1996 PG's use in cat food was banned because it causes a type of anemia that damages hemoglobin.[3] But according to the FDA it's safe for your eats—funny, because it is forbidden in food in Europe (the folks overseas are a little more stringent about what they ingest).

While no long-term research has been done on PG's side effects when consumed in food, a 2010 study published in the *International Journal of Environmental Research and Public Health* revealed that the presence of PG in indoor air (from water-based paints, for example) was associated with asthma, allergies, and sensitization in children.[4] If PG in air can trigger a reaction, could it have some sort of effect when swallowed? Basic logic should tell you that you should run for the hills when you see this ingredient in your food.

Most of the Top-Rated Terminators (TRTs) have GRAS status, while a select few are considered additives by the FDA and require premarket approval. Others are either regulated by other government agencies or *not regulated at all* (as you will learn in the pages ahead). But any way you slice it, the TRTs will forever be controversial among government; food industry (Big Food); industrial agriculture (Big Ag); and the biotech, science, and health communities at large. The message here: Just because the federal government declares an ingredient safe and secure for your precious body doesn't mean that it is.

Now, here's the lowdown on the Top-Rated Terminators so you can start to make educated decisions about what goes in your mouth—a chance to make a difference in your health.

Edible Regulations—Can You Stomach This?

NOT SO SAFE

How the Food and Drug Administration
Lets Food Safety Slip Through the Holes

DETERMINING "SAFETY"
for CHEMICALS in FOOD

A company wants to add a new chemical ingredient to food. Here's the process to establish the ingredient as "safe" and legal to be used in foods.

most companies start here

- or -

OPTION 1

Submit a Food Additive Petition to FDA, with scientific evidence showing the ingredient will be safe for use in food.

FDA reviews the petition, and publishes a notice approving or denying additive status for the ingredient.

IF FDA APPROVES... the company can start using it in food under the terms approved by FDA.

IF FDA DENIES THE PETITION... The substance is considered illegal and may not be used in foods.

OPTION 2

The company makes its own decision that the ingredient is "GRAS" – Generally Recognized As Safe – legal for use in food. The company can notify FDA...

or not. The company can simply start using the ingredient in food.

If the company notifies FDA of its determination that the ingredient is GRAS, FDA will examine the evidence supporting that claim of safety.

OUTCOME 2
FDA raises questions. The company can withdraw its claim that the ingredient is GRAS...

and simply start using the ingredient.

OUTCOME 1
FDA agrees there is sufficient evidence the ingredient is GRAS & legal for use in food.

OUTCOME 3
FDA rejects the claim that the ingredient is safe.

The company can use it in food anyway.

BUT IS IT SAFE?

Why leave it up to the companies to determine whether their own chemical ingredients are safe? Close the loopholes, FDA!

JOIN the CAMPAIGN to STRENGTHEN FDA
bit.ly/GRAS-additives

LEARN which ADDITIVES are SAFE
chemicalcuisine.org

Center for Science in the Public Interest
Source: http://www.fda.gov/food/ingredientspackaginglabeling/gras/default.htm

There are hundreds of substances that go into processed foods without formal approval from the FDA. While you may believe that this federal agency is meticulously monitoring your food, it is not. In other words, companies are typically the ones calling the shots as it relates to an ingredient's safety and its use for consumption. *How the Food and Drug Administration Lets Food Safety Slip Through the Holes* is a wonderful infographic created by Center for Science in the Public Interest (CSPI), a nongovernmental organization (NGO) and consumer advocacy group whose "twin missions are to conduct innovative research and advocacy programs in health and nutrition, and to provide consumers with current, useful information about their health and well-being."[5]

For animals like cattle, pigs, and poultry, the picture is equally as bad, if not worse. A recent report from the Animal Welfare Institute

(AWI), an organization founded in 1951 with the goal of alleviating the suffering of animals caused by people, suggests that claims touting "sustainably produced" on meat and poultry are anything but transparent. After three years of requesting documentation from the USDA from producers touting "Humanely Raised and Handled" to "Sustainably Farmed," the government was unable to provide any proof that these companies were living up to their claims.[6]

The good news is that you can do something about ensuring more stringent food regulations. See Appendix E, "Redeemable Resources," and sign up action alerts from any one of the organizations listed under "Food Policy, Safety, Accountability."

The Terminators

Did you know that people today consume five times more food dye than they did thirty years ago? How about that most artificial vanilla flavoring (including what is found in some bottles of "vanilla" extract) is made from wood pulp? Or that chemical preservatives such as sulfur dioxide, which are commonly used in dried fruit, fruit juices, and molasses, can cause an asthmatic reaction in many? Have you heard about the chemical flavor enhancer MSG (monosodium glutamate)? Although it's been used prevalently in your food supply for more than a hundred years, it can cause *MSG symptom complex*, the symptoms of which include chest pain, difficulty breathing, headache, and nausea.

These are just some of the TRTs. They are pervasive and not going away anytime soon. So if you have any interest in doing better than you are right now when it comes to the foods you choose and your health, it is your job as a consumer to know what the TRTs are, why they are "bad," and what the Better for You Alternatives are, so you can make a conscious choice to consume or avoid.

While there is plenty of science to question the safety of most if not all of the TRTs, there is *not* enough to deem them unsafe for human consumption—meaning a cease-and-desist on their use in anything edible. So full disclosure: Some studies assure us that many of these TRTs (and other foodstuffs) are harmless, but I tend to pay more attention to the studies that raise significant questions about whether consumption can lead to mild to severe health problems. Clearly you know where my bias lies, but look at it this way—why take a risk with your body and your health, or perhaps more important, with that of your loved ones? I prefer to teach my clients how to eat safely. Based on my experience working with people to prevent or manage illness through food, I can honestly tell you that everybody I have worked with feels better after removing (or greatly limiting) the TRTs from the foods they eat. And here's your chance to do the same. While I am by no measure going to hit every "no-no" ingredient in food, let's consider the TRTs—chemical preservatives, artificial flavors and enhancers, artificial colors, artificial sweeteners, sugar and its many euphemisms, trans fats (hydrogenated oils), pesticides, antibiotics, hormones, and genetically modified organisms (GMOs)—a great starting point to reshape your relationship with your eats.

CHAPTER 1

Chemical Preservatives*

Have you ever made your own salad dressing with oil and vinegar, or maybe one with oil, lemon and herbs, and it keeps in the fridge for a couple of weeks? Have you noticed that putting nuts and seeds in the fridge or freezer keeps them longer? What about cookies made from scratch—how long do they keep? A few days out of the cold but much longer in. This is basic food preservation. And edibles can be preserved in many natural ways: packaging (vacuum packs, canning, bottling), storage (in the fridge, in the freezer, and even by burying them in the ground), and preparation methods (drying, smoking, pickling by fermentation, and even pasteurization—the heating of liquid to kill off bacteria).

However, despite the availability of these elementary preservation techniques, the food industry often opts for chemical preservation because it's "safer," it's cheap, and it keeps the "freshness," flavor, color, moisture, and "nutrition" in for longer periods of time. But that's not all—food companies remain profitable if products are shelf stable at room temperature for extensive periods of time. Items can be shipped long distances and sit on market shelves until sold rather than being tossed as soon as they sour.

Businesses have also turned to technology like irradiation (see sidebar, "On Irradiation," page 10) to preserve your eats. Hey, the "safer" the food is and the fresher it looks, the more likely you are to buy it. Time to understand how your eats are kept edible.

*Some are considered Generally Recognized as Safe (GRAS) while others are additives requiring FDA pre-market approval (specifically noted in this chapter).

On Irradiation

According to *Zapped!* by Wenonah Hauter and Mark Worth, "The U.S. is rushing toward food irradiation as the panacea for preventing food poisoning."[1] Industry calls it "cold pasteurization," but I like to refer to it as "X-rayted" food. According to the FDA, irradiation is the application of ionizing radiation to food (waves of energetic particles that change the natural structure of food). Its purpose is not only to prevent food-borne illness as noted, but also to preserve food, prevent insect infestation, and delay sprouting and ripening.

While irradiation appears to neither make food radioactive nor change its nutritional content, the FDA has evaluated its safety for more than thirty years, and the USDA, the Centers for Disease Control and Prevention (CDC), and the World Health Organization (WHO) all give it a thumbs-up; however, its use on edibles is highly controversial.

Zapped! is an exposé on irradiation, and the long and short of it is that there is substantial evidence in multiple peer-reviewed journals (the place where you go for the scientific facts) to question the true safety of this innovative preservation process. For example, in 1975 the *American Journal of Clinical Nutrition*'s "Effects of Feeding Irradiated Wheat to Malnourished Children" reported that after fifteen children were fed freshly irradiated wheat, they developed abnormal cells in growing number as the feeding duration increased. While the *biological significance* of abnormal cells was not fully understood, its association with malignancy suggested that consumption of irradiated wheat be *fully assessed*.[2]

But let's get real: The contamination of food is not something that irradiation will be able to solve—more stringent food safety rules and regulations are in order.

Despite debate concerning the safety of irradiation, some foods are approved for irradiation in the United States, including the following:

- Beef and pork
- Poultry
- Molluscan shellfish (oysters, clams, mussels, and scallops)
- Shell eggs
- Fresh fruit and vegetables
- Lettuce and spinach
- Spices and seasonings
- Seeds for sprouting (such as alfalfa sprouts)

While the FDA requires that irradiated food have the international symbol for irradiation—the Radura (see the figure)—with the statement "Treated with radiation" or "Treated by irradiation" on the label, foods that *contain* irradiated ingredients *do not* need to be labeled. This is alarming considering the fact that roughly 10 percent of herbs and spices in the United States are irradiated, so whether your food has the Radura on it or not, there is still a lack of transparency as to whether it contains irradiated ingredients.

Radura symbol

For the moment, the only way to truly confirm that your food is not irradiated is to know what's in the irradiation wheelhouse and to opt into organics where you can. That is, if you feel as suspect about irradiation as I do.

What Preservatives Are and Why They Are "Bad"

By definition, food preservation is the process of treating and handling food to stop or slow down spoilage, loss of quality, edibility, or nutritional value, thus allowing for longer food storage.

Chemical preservatives—the antimicrobials that stop the green stuff from growing, and the antioxidants that prevent oxidation (the chemical reaction between oxygen and food that cause spoilage)—could very well promote illness. So pick and choose wisely.

Take a peek in your pantry, fridge, and even freezer—from the can of soup to the trusted tortillas, the hummus to the Ho Hos; most likely, somewhere on each product's ingredient list, you will see one of the following chemical preservatives. Yes, preservatives are necessary to keep your food safe, but there are better ways to go about it than to use these synthetics (more on this later).

ANTIMICROBIALS

Benzoates (GRAS)

Sodium benzoate (and its close relative benzoic acid) has been used in food manufacturing for a century to prevent the growth of microorganisms in acidic foods such as fruit juice, carbonated drinks, and pickles. While benzoates occur naturally in many plants and animals and appear to be safe for most people, they can cause hives, asthma, or other allergic reactions in sensitive individuals.

Apparently when sodium benzoate is used in beverages that also contain ascorbic acid (vitamin C) like fruit juices, the two substances can react to form small amounts of benzene—a chemical that has been linked to leukemia and other cancers. While the amounts of formed benzene are small, leading to a minute risk of cancer, in the 1990s the FDA urged companies to eliminate the use of benzoate in products that also contain ascorbic acid, but they didn't want to listen. So in 2006, a private attorney filed a lawsuit that in the end forced Coca-Cola, PepsiCo, and other U.S. soft-drink companies to reformulate beverages of concern—typically the fruit-flavored products. Even still, Dr Pepper cherry and Schweppes Ginger Ale, compliments of Dr Pepper Snapple Group, remains unchanged.[3]

Sorbates (GRAS)

Potassium sorbate is commonly used to prevent the growth of mold in cheese, baked goods including breads and tortillas, dried fruit, jelly, syrups, and wine. Most research deems this as one of the least offensive chemical preservatives, but a study published in 2010 in *Toxicology in Vitro*[4] showed that potassium sorbate was toxic to human DNA in a type of white blood cell. In other words, this additive could affect your immunity. Given that potassium sorbate is one of the most common antimicrobials, watch what you eat.

Sulfites (GRAS)

You've heard this term used in reference to wine (see sidebar, "On Wine and Sulfites," page 14). Yes, sulfites occur naturally, to some extent, in vino, but nonnatural versions like potassium bisulfite, potassium metabisulfite, sodium bisulfite, sodium metabisulfite, sodium sulfite, and their close relative sulfur dioxide are added to your eats to keep your food fresh. And while most of you may not notice a darn thing when you consume them (in foods such as cookies, crackers, pizza crust, and tortillas; dried fruit, whether solo or in trail mixes; condiments and relishes; sugar derived from sugar beets; molasses; fresh or frozen shrimp and lobster; canned clams; gelatins, puddings, and fillers; jams and jellies; shredded coconut; processed vegetables— canned, pickled, instant, or frozen; dried soup mixes; syrups including corn and maple; and citrus juice concentrates, instant tea and alcoholic beverages including beer, wine, wine coolers, and mixers), the FDA estimates that one out of one hundred people have some form of sensitivity to sulfites.

Reactions can include sneezing, swelling of the throat, trouble breathing, and even anaphylactic shock in the most extreme cases. That's enough to make me want to stay away whenever possible, especially given the fact that reacting to sulfites can blindside you—it can happen at any given time despite the fact that you may have been okay with those bright orange dried apricots (that are only neon because of the sulfites) your whole life.

Sadly, regulations on sulfites are weak. Seafood often contains sulfites and while labeling is required, it is not well enforced (more on this in sidebar "A Fishy Situation," page 80). In 1986, the FDA did ban the use of sulfites in foods intended to be eaten fresh, like fruits and vegetables (salad bars should technically be safe now), but food managers are not required to disclose whether sulfites were used during food preparation (for example, to keep potatoes fresh before cooking). The good news is that when sulfites are used as a preservative in packaged foods, they must be listed on the label if *above* 10 parts per million. Even so, according to the FDA, "any standardized food that, as a result of actions that are consistent with current good manufacturing practice, contains an indirectly added sulfiting agent that has no functional effect, [the chemical] is considered to be an incidental additive."[5] In other words, no labeling is required. Any way you slice it, sulfites are sneaking into your food without your knowing it.

On Wine and Sulfites

While sulfites do occur naturally in wine as a by-product of fermentation, they are also added to wine in their chemical form to prevent spoilage—mostly to lighter wines like whites and rosés. In the United States, organic wines typically don't have any added sulfites; there are also some sulfur-free wines on the market, but in order to make them, the sulfites are typically chemically removed with hydrogen peroxide. If you have a reaction to sulfites, simply avoid wine.

Sodium Nitrates and Sodium Nitrites
(additive; subject to premarket approval by FDA)

While fresh vegetables naturally contain nitrates (that convert to nitrites in your saliva), their chemical counterparts are used to preserve cured foods like bacon, hot dogs, jerky, lunch meats, and some smoked foods like salmon. Both sodium nitrate and sodium nitrite prevent bacterial growth and help keep the color and flavor in. According to the World Cancer Research Fund and the American Institute for Cancer Research, consumption of processed meats is linked to increased risk of colorectal cancer. Nitrosamine, a known carcinogen, forms when nitrates and nitrites marry with protein-rich foods like meats.[6] Many companies are starting to opt out of these chemical additions (a good thing). Even so, they are still ever-present in the marketplace. Please do your best to avoid these likely noxious nitrates and nitrites.

ANTIOXIDANTS

Butylated Hydroxyanisole (BHA) and Butylated Hydroxytoluene (BHT) (GRAS)

BHA (which is typically accompanied by BHT in processed foods) retards rancidity in fats, oils, and oil-containing foods. This chemical is often found in cereals, chewing gum, potato chips, and vegetable oil, and its use is highly controversial. While no adequate human studies have been conducted, the consumption of BHA by rats, mice, and hamsters has a strong relationship with cancer. According to the National Institutes of Health, the specific cancers occurred in the forestomach, an organ that humans do not have.

However, according to CSPI, a chemical that causes cancer in at least one organ in three different species indicates that it might be carcinogenic in humans.[7] That is why the U.S. Department of Health and Human Services considers BHA "reasonably anticipated to be a human carcinogen."[8] Nevertheless, the FDA still permits BHA in your food. When it comes to BHT (often found in the same foods as BHA), continuous debate surrounds its direct link to cancer, as only some studies suggest an increased risk of the big C while others refute it. The reality is that BHT typically goes hand in hand with BHA, so I would just steer clear of the butylated buddies.

Propyl Gallate (GRAS)

While not a super-popular additive anymore, propyl gallate is often used in conjunction with BHA and BHT to stave off rancidity in oils and fats. When used, it is found in meat products, microwave popcorn, soup mixes, chewing gum, mayonnaise, and frozen meals. While the FDA considers propyl gallate safe for consumption, a 1982 study conducted by the National Toxicology Program of the U.S. Department of Health and Human Services noted that this chemical can cause malignancy in mice and rats.[9] And according to the CSPI's Chemical Cuisine,* an online guide to food additives, propyl gallate should be avoided.[10]

Tert-Butylhydroquinone (TBHQ) (additive; subject to premarket approval by FDA)

Supposedly TBHQ is safe. Often found alongside the other antioxidants—BHA, BHT, and propyl gallate—this chemical rears its head in many oily fast foods like McDonald's chicken nuggets[11] as well as some common baked goods and cereals. Basically, the safety of TBHQ is dependent on length of exposure and consumption levels; over time it is thought to damage DNA and possibly cause cancer. And while most people won't down enough TBHQ in one sitting to have lasting effects, its subtle presence in many foods and the danger of persistent intake should make you wary.

The Better for You Alternatives

Let's get back to basics. As I mentioned, before chemical unspoilers were created, food preservation was simply done with packaging, storage, and preparation methods that required salt, acid, or sugar. There are also plenty

---

*For more extensive and regularly updated information on these chemicals and many others including what is listed in *What the Fork*, visit cspinet.org/reports/chemcuisine.htm.

of safer options now available, including ascorbic acid (vitamin C) and its derivatives such as sodium erythorbate, erythobic acid, and sodium isoascorbate; alpha tocopherol (vitamin E); and naturally occurring citric acid—all of which are listed as such on labels today.

Although it is preferable to consume fresh food or food simply preserved with salt, acid, or sugar, food processing sometimes demands more than that. I get that you probably can't avoid packaged foods (hey, I can't 100 percent either), so try to do what I do—pick and choose wisely to avoid the more offensive chemicals and aim for some of the safer options mentioned here, which can be found in everything from cereal to boxed meals to snack foods today.

CHAPTER 2

Artificial Flavors and Enhancers*

Have you ever wondered what it means when a product says it is "artificially flavored"? Even "naturally flavored"? There are roughly ten large flavor companies worldwide (as well as many smaller ones) that shape the story of your food, and believe it or not, the New Jersey Turnpike runs through the heart of this industry, serving up roughly 70 percent of the manufactured food flavor in the United States.

When a food is processed to the extent you see in packaged products, the natural flavors are largely lost. Thus a small handful of elite flavorists come up with tasty chemical concoctions that make your food—ranging from Kellogg's Pop-Tarts to Nature's Path organic Toaster Pastries—worth eating. You will never know what is actually in these flavors, as the "recipes" are proprietary. I call the world of flavoring the "food CIA"—we know these flavor companies are up to something, but we never really know what it is. To give you an idea, roughly sixty-three flavor agents are used to create the artificial strawberry flavor found in a Burger King "strawberry" milk shake. And for natural flavors, the picture doesn't look much different.

A couple of years ago, a small group of people came to me asking for a third-party nutrition review of a food product they wanted to bring to market. The CEO said, "I know you will keep us honest." Well, after reviewing their product, I had many questions like, "What comprises your 'natural' flavors?" Very determined to get some answers, they cautiously connected

*Considered Generally Recognized as Safe (GRAS).

me with their flavor company's food scientist. And this is what I found out: There were roughly twenty-plus compounds in the "natural" flavor, but the food scientist would *not* reveal their sources other than that they were derived from something "natural." Of course I wanted to know more, but he offered nothing. In fact, he evaded the remainder of my questions, including those that concerned the source of many other ingredients and the true process of how the product was being made. My take: There is an unspoken "Processed Food Privacy Act"—a code of honor among food and beverage makers that keeps edible creations clandestine. Most of the people making your food really don't want to tell you how they do it because if they did, you probably wouldn't buy it. It's typically about their bottom line, not your health. So my advice to the CEO was, if you want to create a reputable product for consumption, you want transparency from your team. And you will not get it from these flavor savers.

What They Are

According to an article published in *Scientific American* in 2002, there is little substantive difference in the chemical compositions of natural and artificial flavorings—they are both made in a laboratory by elite flavorists and their many favored food scientists. "Natural" chemicals are used to make natural flavorings, and "synthetic" chemicals make artificial flavorings.[1] The distinction between natural versus artificial comes from the *source* of these chemicals. For example (and quite simply put), natural vanilla flavor is derived from the vanilla bean itself, while artificial vanilla flavor comes from synthetic chemicals whose origin is unrelated to food (as in wood or even cow poop—more on that later).

According to the FDA's Code of Federal Regulations, the term "natural flavor" or "natural flavoring" means the "Essential oil, oleoresin (mixture of essential oils and resin), essence of extractive, protein hydrolysate, distillate or any product of roasting, heating, or enzymolysis [a tongue twister but basically means breaking down with a little help from something natural] which contains the flavoring constituents derived from a spice, fruit or fruit juice, vegetable or vegetable juice, edible yeast, herb, bark, bud, root, leaf or similar plant material, meat, seafood, poultry, eggs, dairy products, or fermentation products thereof, whose significant function in food is flavoring rather than nutritional."

In contrast, the Code of Federal Regulations defines the term "artificial flavor" or "artificial flavoring" as "Any substance used to impart flavor that is *not* derived from a spice, fruit or fruit juice, vegetable or vegetable juice, edible yeast, herb, bark, bud, root, leaf or similar plant material, meat, seafood, poultry, eggs, dairy products, or fermentation products thereof."[2]

Now that you are clear on the difference between natural and artificial flavors, it is important to know that distinct chemical components from both sources are what flavor your food. And it is often the marriage of many of these chemicals that makes food taste good. So whether you are eating an apple or drinking apple juice with natural flavors or artificial ones, the same basic chemicals are giving your eats their edibleness.

Why They Are "Bad"

I am not going to vilify natural flavors, but I will tell you this—they are concocted in a lab, and you will never know their true sources or how the actual flavors are derived from their "naturalness." So I do have questions about them in general, and so should you. As Eric Schlosser so poignantly states in his *New York Times* bestseller *Fast Food Nation*, "Natural and artificial flavors are now manufactured at the same chemical plants, places that few people would associate with Mother Nature. Calling any of these flavors 'natural' requires a flexible attitude toward the English language and a fair amount of irony."[3]

As far as artificial flavors are concerned, I just don't go there. In 2006, Mayu Yamamoto, a former researcher at the International Medical Center of Japan, won the Ig Nobel Prize (a parody of the Nobel Prize, granted by the *Annals of Improbable Research*, a science humor magazine, that is "meant to make people laugh and then think") for developing a technique for extracting vanillin—the chemical in a vanilla bean that gives it its distinct flavor—from cow poop.[4] She received her award at Harvard University in 2007 and had this to say: "At first I thought it was a joke, but came to the award ceremony hoping my research would become more widely known."[5] She suggested that widespread adoption of her method could help the environment—it would give companies a use for cow poop, which contributes to global warming. Seriously, I get the global warming thing and doing all that you can to create a sustainable environment, but what the fork? Human beings should be eating real food—as in vanilla derived from vanilla beans, not dung. While you won't find fake vanilla from poop in your food today, maybe someday you will.

So folks, you will never know what is truly in your flavorings, whether natural or artificial, what they are *truly* derived from, how they are derived, and whether the chemicals combined to make your food taste so good are actually safe because the U.S. government accepts these concoctions as "generally recognized as safe," meaning that they are perfectly fine (based on loose evidence or long-term use without concern), until they are *not*.

The Better for You Alternatives

Let's face it: Food flavorings are unavoidable for most, even me. I do eat some processed foods with "natural" flavors, as do my kids. But doing it cautiously is the key. Seeking foods *without* that ambiguous "natural flavors" at the tail end of the ingredient list is the way to go. Otherwise, it just feels too CIA for me. I look for specific ingredients like "strawberry juice," "blueberry essence," or "pure vanilla extract" on the label, which makes me a little more comfy with my choices.

While buying packaged food with the artificials is cheaper all around, healthier brands are becoming widely available these days; as I always say, do you want to pay on the front end or the back end? You have that choice. Sticking with fresh food is ideal, but hey, everyone needs a little pro-cessed "goodness" in their lives.

Speaking of which, it's good to know that Annie's—the Kraft Foods for the conscious eater, which makes everything from frozen pizza and maca-roni and cheese to crackers and other snack foods—rarely uses "natural" flavorings. Rather, the taste of their products is supported by real-food ingredients like cheese, herbs, and spices.

On the Flavor Enhancer Monosodium Glutamate (MSG) (GRAS)

While I was watching a popular Food Network show, the featured chef was making homemade empanadas (Spanish stuffed bread that looks like a calzone). To my utter astonishment, he tossed MSG—a white granular synthetic chemical that is used as a flavor enhancer—into his commercial-size mixer while making *fresh dough*. What the Fork? Typi-cally found in Chinese restaurant food whether dining in or taking out, fast food, and processed foods from soups and sauces to lunch meats and snacks, MSG is thought to improve the overall taste of food.

According to the Mayo Clinic, numerous anecdotal reports show that MSG causes adverse reactions in many. These reactions include head-ache; flushing; sweating; facial pressure or tightness; numbness, tingling, or burning in the face, neck, and other areas; rapid, fluttering heartbeats (like palpitations); chest pain; nausea; and weakness. However, there are no large-scale data to prove that MSG is unsafe for consumption.[6]

Monosodium glutamate is typically listed on labels if it's an ingredient in your food. While it used to fall under "spices" or "flavorings," meaning that you would never know whether your product contained MSG, in 1998 that all changed—it had to stand alone on labels because of its ill effects on many. However, do be wary of Chinese food and fast food as there is no transparency there unless you ask—so questioning what's in your grub when you go out to eat is a must.

CHAPTER 3

Artificial Colors*

A few summers ago, my friend's son David was selling lemonade on Main Street for charity. I took my oldest boy, Jack, then four, into town to contribute to the cause. Now, I must preface this by saying that Jack has been in the kitchen with me since he was old enough to sit in a high-chair, and I have been talking to him about food—the good, the bad, and the ugly.

As we pulled up we noticed that not only was David selling lemonade, but he was also drinking red Gatorade. Well, Jack took one look at him, put his little hands on his hips, and said, "That drink has Red No. 40 in it, and if you drink it, you will get sick."

David, who is four years older than Jack, had fear in his eyes. "What is Red No. 40?"

Jack turned to me. "Take it from here, Mom." I was so proud of my little nutrition know-it-all.

What They Are

Today, the FDA defines a color additive as any "dye, pigment, or other substance that can impart color to a food, drug, or cosmetic or to the human body."[1]

---

*Considered additives and require premarket approval.

In 1856, English chemist William Henry Perkin derived the color mauve from coal tar—the thick black liquid produced by the distillation of coal—marking the beginning of the story of synthetic dyes, first for fabric, then for food. But today many artificial colorings come from petroleum—a naturally occurring flammable liquid that is found in rock formations beneath the earth's surface. So, the same chemical building blocks that were once extracted from coal tar to make food dye are now being pulled from petroleum because it's cheaper and more plentiful and efficient (not as messy as coal tar).

Sadly, fake colors have been favored over their natural plant-based counterparts like paprika or beet juice because artificial colors cost less, are more stable, and much brighter. Their ultimate purpose is to keep your food vibrant—whether to compensate for color lost during processing, correct natural variations in color, enhance existing color, or provide radiance to otherwise colorless products that need to be *fun*, like candy. Artificial colors are classified as *straights* (single dyes that are not mixed with another substance), *lakes* (straights that are mixed with aluminum to make the dye more dispersible and that are often found in cake and doughnut mixes, candy, and gum), and *mixtures* (the marriage of multiple straights that can be found in confections like candy).

Unlike many other common food additives, dyes require premarket approval by the FDA. According to the agency, "by 1900, many foods, drugs and cosmetics available in the United States were artificially colored. However, *not all* coloring agents *were harmless* and some were being used to hide inferior or defective foods. In many cases, the toxicities of the starting materials for synthesizing coloring agents were well known and could be toxins, irritants, sensitizers or carcinogens."[2]

While the regulators were busy questioning and scrutinizing the colors, people continued to get sick. In 1950, many children fell ill after eating orange Halloween candy containing 1–2 percent Orange No. 1—a color that had been approved for use. This event, as well as concerns at the time regarding the carcinogenicity of food additives, prompted the FDA to think twice about the colors; lo and behold, they found that several caused health problems. The rainbow was fading. According to the FDA, the Color Additives Amendment of 1960 finally defined "color additive" and made certain that only color additives listed as suitable and safe for a given use could be used in foods, drugs, and cosmetics. The FDA revamped their procedural regulations for approval, and roughly two hundred colors in use were temporarily listed and could be used only on an interim basis until their use was banned due to safety concerns or lack of industrial interest or they were deemed permissible because of their known "safety."

Today, about one hundred dyes are still listed for use by the FDA, and according to the Center for Science in the Public Interest, nine dyes are approved for use in food, drugs, and cosmetics. But just *three* of the nine dyes—Red No. 40, Yellow No. 5, and Yellow No. 6—account for 90 percent of all dyes used. Americans have come to expect a rainbow of colors in such foods as candy, soda, cereals, snacks, baked goods, frozen foods, and condiments. Dyes can even be found in foods you don't expect—many jarred pickles actually have Yellow No. 5 in them even though there are plenty on the market that do just fine without the added color. U.S. consumption of food dye has increased fivefold since 1955, according to the CSPI.[3] And you have paid the price.

Why They Are "Bad"

Over the years, many dyes have been banned because of their adverse effects on lab animals. This rainbow of colors comes with significant levels of risk—enough that in 2008, the European Food Safety Authority required that all foods containing dyes have warning labels, prompting many companies to move away from the dyes and go with natural sources of coloring. So a McDonald's strawberry sundae in Europe gets its color from strawberries, but in the United States, it gets its color from Red No. 40. Go figure.

Why did the European Food Safety Authority require those labels? Because studies have shown that these dyes trigger allergies, cause hyperactivity in children, and can even lead to cancer. In fact, the labels alone prompted many corporations, from McDonald's to Coca-Cola (orange Fanta is now dye-free in Europe), to rethink how they were making their food. But not in this country.

When confirming that an additive is safe to eat, testing should be done in long-term animal feeding studies conducted by a third party. But sadly, this is typically not the case. Trials that measure the safety of a foodstuff are often short-term and funded by the company making the product—so in the end, where is the objectivity? According to the CSPI's extensive report "Food Dyes: A Rainbow of Risks,"* which was released in 2009, there are many causes for concern.[4]

CARCINOGENICITY (CAUSING CANCER)

Interestingly, dyes are not pure chemicals—they contain roughly 10 percent impurities. For example, benzidine—a known human carcinogen that as of 2012 was listed in the Environmental Protection Agency's *Chemicals of Concern* (a list of chemicals that require action to reduce exposure)—is a common adulterant in the compounds used to make food dyes. While the FDA has established legal limits for these contaminants and those limits are *supposed* to ensure that these artificial colors will cause cancer in *only* one in one million people (which is still too many, as far as I am concerned), these tolerances were based on dye usage in 1990. Since then, usage has drastically increased (as mentioned previously). In addition, the FDA never considered the risk to children, who not only consume more dye per unit of body weight than adults but also are more sensitive to carcinogens.

GENOTOXICITY (CAUSING GENE MUTATIONS OR DAMAGE)

Think of your body as a house. All houses start with a blueprint, and the blueprint for all living organisms, including you, is your DNA. From these information molecules, your genes—a carefully coded copy of a small part

---

*For more extensive information on food dyes, visit cspinet.org/new/pdf/food-dyes-rainbow-of-risks.pdf.

of your DNA—are made. For the purpose of the house analogy, let's look at these genes as very specific instructions on how to build your house, from where the rooms go to the color of the walls.

Certain chemicals can cause mutations or damage to your DNA, precipitating problems within your genes (those house-building instructions). If your body is injured at the gene level, your cells can be abnormal—and abnormal cells are at the root of many cancers today. (This will make a fragile house).

So what do dyes have to do with genes? Several animal studies need to be conducted to determine the safety of foodstuffs. Ideally, all (or most) studies should come back negative—meaning that the chemical being tested is "safe." Let's take Yellow No. 5 as an example; out of the eleven studies conducted on this dye's safety, six of the studies came back showing genotoxicity, according to CSPI's report. That's pretty alarming, considering that Yellow No. 5 is the second most widely used dye, found in everything from pickles to pastries.

Thus, if you are genotoxic, your genes are likely damaged. These altered genes produce abnormal cells and other mutations that can be the precursor to a spectrum of illnesses. In addition, these damaged genes can be passed down to children without their ever being directly exposed to the toxin.

NEUROTOXICITY (CAUSING NEUROLOGICAL DAMAGE)

The relationship between food dyes and neurotoxicity is still disputed. In 1973, Dr. Benjamin Feingold, a pediatric allergist from California, proposed that certain food additives, including food dyes, cause hyperactivity in children and even adults. He created the Feingold Diet—a food elimination program that removes dyes, along with a number of other artificial ingredients, from a person's diet. While mainstream medical wisdom dismissed his work, stating that it lacked scientific evidence, his findings generated quite a bit of publicity. It motivated many scientists to study the cause-and-effect relationship between food dyes and hyperactivity. And in 2004, a study published in the *Journal of Developmental and Behavioral*

Pediatrics by David Schab and Nhi-Ha T. Trinh concluded that dyes promote hyperactivity in "hyperactive" children, legitimizing the call for a broader discussion about the use of food dyes.[5]

The Better for You Alternatives

It turns out that my friend's son David no longer drinks red Gatorade. He has other choices, and so do you. There is now a dye-free version of Gatorade, as well as other sports drinks (or various quenchers) without fake color. If you are looking for the perfect hydrator for the active lifestyle, opt for one of my favorite electrolyte-packed bevvies—coconut water. Also check out ElectroMIX powder from the makers of Emergen-C to add some nutrients and fizz to your H_2O. Choose foods without dyes (you now know what to look out for). Believe it or not, everything from Froot Loops to Fun Dip has a not-so-evil twin that is colored with natural dyes derived from fruits, vegetables, herbs, and spices, including berries, beets, annatto (though some are sensitive to it), and paprika. In fact, you can even buy natural food dyes from India Tree—although they are more costly and not widely available in stores—to color your cookies and cakes. Oh, and if you are the sort to color your kids' eggs à la *Green Eggs and Ham*, purée a little spinach, and you've got your green plus some extra nutrition.

CHAPTER 4

Artificial Sweeteners*

This is just priceless! Artificial sweeteners were discovered in 1878 by a researcher working out of a lab at Johns Hopkins who noticed that a derivative of coal tar he accidentally spilled on his hand tasted sweet. His spill set the stage for the development of saccharin—the first artificial sweetener introduced to market. Sadly, saccharin and other seriously sweet substances are granted GRAS status by the FDA despite incredible controversy.

As a result of studies conducted in the 1970s that linked saccharin to cancer in lab rats, saccharin once carried a warning label that said consumption could be hazardous to your health. But apparently it is now in the clear, as newer studies have "confirmed" its safety (more on this later). Scientifically speaking, *nothing is wrong with this chemical despite the fact that multiple studies have linked it to cancer in rodents.*

While I can't compare all artificial sweeteners to saccharin, as they're not all created "equal" (though they are all seriously chemicalized), I like to look at a lot more than the science when making food choices.

Marion Nestle, PhD, MPH, one of the most notable experts in the debate over the safety and health of the American food system, looks at two distinct factors in assessing risky eats in her book *Safe Food*. You can evaluate edibles from a science-based perspective (calculating illness by its frequency and severity, benefits of risk, and cost of the risk) and from a

*Most are considered Generally Recognized as Safe (GRAS) (specifically noted in chapter).

value-based point of view (determining whether the risk is voluntary or imposed, understood or uncertain, natural or technological).[1] I trust science. But when it comes to things in your food or being done to your food, the science can be highly subjective (depending on who is funding the research, who truly benefits from the use of those ingredients or processes, and if enough hard evidence exists to determine the true safety for human consumption and the environment).

According to Nestle, "In 1979 Philip Handler, then president of the National Academy of Sciences said that the *estimation* of risk is a scientific question—and, therefore a legitimate activity of scientists in federal agencies, in universities and the National Research Council. The *acceptability* of a given level of risk, however, is a political question to be determined by the political arena."[2]

Hey, what about the consumer? Don't you have a say about what goes in your food? By now you are probably catching on to the fact that food regulation is pretty much a free-for-all.

So maybe from a science-based perspective, saccharin and its crappy cousins are "safe," but from a value-based point of view, do you honestly think that consuming something so artificial can support health in any way whatsoever? You eat it because it makes your food sweet (anywhere from thirty to eight thousand times sweeter than sugar) *without* the calories—one gram of table sugar contains four calories, while these artificial heroes have zero. Consequently, for a sugar- and calorie-obsessed nation, it is the perfect panacea—you can eat all the sweets you want without taking in any calories.

I know, you are probably thinking that these sweeteners are medically necessary for many—like the 25.8 million Americans living with diabetes (90 to 95 percent of whom have type 2 diabetes, also called adult-onset diabetes)[3] or the grossly overweight and obese population. Well, this is what you are made to believe, but the reality is that if you are diagnosed with diabetes, eating all the same stuff with artificial sweetness is not going to help; changing your diet and adding exercise to your routine will. While I am vehemently opposed to every single fake sweetener, I get that many of you embrace them. My goal is to meet you where you are at, but at the same time push you to do a little better. So I beg you to try to limit your intake of anything chemically sweet—as you will read next, most of them are *highly* questionable.

What They Are and Why They Are "Bad"

According to the Mayo Clinic, artificial sweeteners are sugar substitutes whose sweetness comes from chemically manufactured molecules that *do not* exist in nature.[4] These molecules are manipulated in a lab to give you one of the five zero-calorie-won't-raise-your-blood-sugar phonies that have GRAS status as per the FDA and are embraced by the food industry and consumers at large.

Since artificial sweeteners are everywhere, I won't even attempt to list all of the places they live, but let me offer a clue: Anything that says "light," "low sugar," "reduced sugar," "no added sugar," "zero calories," or "calorie-free" is probably laden with one or more of the following. You can find them in food and beverages; in the sugar/baking aisle in any grocery store; and let's not forget the small packets on the tables of coffee shops and eateries to sweeten your tea, cup of joe, or whatever else you fancy.

SACCHARIN (AKA SWEET'N LOW, SWEET TWIN, AND NECTA SWEET) (GRAS)

The sneaky little history of saccharin stinks as far as I am concerned. As it is the very first superficial sweetener and is now considered one of the most studied additives in your food supply, its journey into and out of and back into your eats is notable.

Saccharin was introduced in the 1880s, and by 1908, Harvey Wiley, the head of the USDA's Bureau of Chemistry (which would later be known as the Food and Drug Administration) proposed the first saccharin ban—how could a coal tar derivative be safe for human consumption? But because of inconclusive scientific evidence, this chemical remained in the food supply. Haven't we heard this story before? Although saccharin was considered harmless in small doses, it was finally prohibited in foods in July 1912 because consumers would ingest more than a "small dose" over the course of their lives. This ban was upheld for years because of a "bureaucratic stalemate between regulators and industry," according to the Chemical Heritage Foundation, an organization that fosters an understanding of chemistry's impact on society.[5]

Speaking of industry, saccharin was one of biochemical giant Monsanto Company's first consumer products (more on this later). When World War I caused a sugar shortage (leading to an increase in sugar prices), Monsanto flexed its muscles and went to the public with full-page ads making the case that saccharin could save the country millions of dollars. Money-minded consumers responded and bought into the saccharin scam. When the war ended, the nation was back to sugar—but not for long, as World War II was met with the same shortage, and saccharin was there to save the day. After World War II, Americans (becoming increasingly concerned with their waistlines) continued to embrace saccharin as it made its way back into the food supply in the many processed foods that permeated grocery store shelves.

The nation's consumption of this inexpensive, no-calorie sweetener was on the rise, and nutritionists and health officials became alarmed—the debate over its safety was still not settled.

In 1958, the Delaney Clause, an amendment to the Food, Drug, and Cosmetic Act of 1938, required that "The Secretary of the Food and Drug Administration shall not approve for use in food any chemical additive found to induce cancer in man, or, after tests, found to induce cancer in animals."[6]

But as science advanced and chemicals became more widely used in foods, regulatory agencies were challenged to the core by the food industry. There was a loophole in the Delaney Clause making it possible to put cancer-causing chemicals in your food in *really small concentrations* (1 part per million). In other words, Delaney didn't fully address quantification and risk assessment for potential carcinogens. So that *really small* quantity has been and continues to be presumed "safe" for human consumption (until it is *not*).

Right around the time Delaney took a stance, Sweet'N Low was introduced to the market. This pink packet of poison was a mixture of saccharin, cyclamate (another fake that is now passé), and other ingredients like anticaking agents and was ever-so-present in diners and coffee shops across the country. Plus in the 1960s diet soda was in. However, in the late sixties, cyclamate was banned because of its link to cancer. And then around 1970, one study pointed to a possible link between increased bladder cancer in rats that consumed saccharin daily.[7] Thus in 1972 the FDA attempted to ban saccharin. However, Monsanto and the rest of the sugar-free-loving food industry fought hard with "counterevidence" and megamedia campaigns to keep this potentially cancer-causing criminal out of jail. And eventually they won, but foods with this chemical would have to wear a warning label. By 2000, labeling was deemed unnecessary because there was *supposedly* no longer anything to worry about (despite saccharin's on-and-off relationship with the Environmental Protection Agency's "black-list"). So while saccharin (whether in packets bearing the names Sweet'N Low, Sweet Twin, or Necta Sweet or as a standalone ingredient in processed foods) is widely adored and consumed by millions, questions still remain about its true safety.

ASPARTAME (AKA NUTRASWEET, EQUAL, AND SUGAR TWIN) (GRAS)

In 1981, the FDA approved the use of aspartame in foods meant for dieting, including beverages, drink mixes, and all types of desserts. Although the use of aspartame is widely accepted worldwide, there is much cause for concern.

Dr. John Olney, a noted medical doctor and professor of psychiatry, pathology, and immunology at Washington University School of Medicine, is well known for his work on brain damage. He has been studying aspartame since the 1970s, and based on his findings that aspartame destroys nerve cells in the brains of mice, he protested the approval of the chemical sweetener in the early eighties and was granted a hearing by the FDA. Despite scientific evidence, his concerns, and those of other noted scientists, the use of aspartame in food was approved in 1981. The reason? The FDA claims lack of effective evidence, *but*, dear readers, the sad truth is that the government is often in cahoots with industry and often officials leave their jobs to work with the companies that are "poisoning" your food (and vice versa). In 1996, Olney published "Increasing Brain Tumor Rates: Is There a Link to Aspartame?" in the *Journal of Neuropathology and Experimental Neurology* and concluded that there was a need to "reassess the carcinogenic potential of aspartame."[8]

As noted by the CSPI, independent scientists have been pressured over the years to conduct new animal studies to further investigate the aspartame-cancer connection. In 2005, the Ramazzini Foundation in Bologna, Italy, conducted that first study indicating that rats exposed to aspartame beginning at eight weeks old through their lifetime developed lymphomas, leukemias, and other tumors.[9] In 2007, the same researchers published a follow-up study in which they had exposed rats to aspartame in utero. That study, too, found that aspartame caused leukemias and lymphomas as well as mammary (breast) cancer.[10] Then in 2010, they studied mice that had been exposed to aspartame in utero forward; that study found that aspartame caused liver and lung cancer in males.[11]

Basically the FDA and the European Food Safety Authority have ignored these findings, noting that the studies were seriously flawed (including, but not limited to, the varied age of the rats being studied and methodology of data collection). The CSPI and other scientists have found these allegations to be meritless and offer this: "The bottom line is that three independent studies have found that consumption of aspartame causes cancer in rodents. That should be reason enough for the FDA (and other governments) to eliminate aspartame from the food supply."[12] Sadly, aspartame and its use in foods around the world is here to stay (for the moment).

ACESULFAME-K (AKA ACESULFAME POTASSIUM, ACE K, SUNETT, AND SWEET ONE) (GRAS)

You've heard the story before: This calorie-free sugar substitute was discovered by a scientist working in a lab with chemicals. After accidentally dipping his fingers in the compounds he was working with, Karl Clauss proceeded to lick his digits to pick up a piece of paper, and lo and behold, he tasted something sweet. This set the stage for further research into what you now see as an ingredient in many processed foods claiming to be "sugar-free," "zero calories," or the like or branded as Sunett or Sweet One. Prior to 1998, acesulfame-K was permitted only in sugar-free baked goods, gum, and gelatin desserts like Jell-O. Then the FDA permitted its use in soft drinks as well.

According to the CSPI, the safety tests conducted in the 1970s were less than adequate. Either they were too brief, rendering them incomplete, or animals were not tested while pregnant (to understand the effects of the chemical on a fetus). Also, two studies did suggest possible carcinogenicity. Despite the lack of evidence, possible carcinogenicity, and the efforts of the CSPI to urge the FDA to do more testing before opening the floodgates, the U.S. government let it rip. Now this artificial sweetener is everywhere. It even partners with sucralose (Splenda) in many "sugar-free" products. As the CSPI says, "Hopefully the small amounts [of Acesulfame-K] in food are not harmful, but it needs to be better tested."[13]

SUCRALOSE (AKA SPLENDA) (GRAS)

From Splenda's website: "As the legend goes, researchers from an established British college were trying out a new compound made from sugar, called sucralose, when a young scientist misheard a request to *test* it as an ask to *taste* it. They discovered it was sweet, but that wasn't even the best part! Sucralose was not only deliciously sweet but also calorie-free! And although it wasn't sugar, it was still good for cooking and baking. At this moment, a healthier way to sweeten was born."[14]

So a synthetic sweetener is healthier than the real stuff? The Splenda story continues in that small-town mom-and-pop-discovery tone, so by the end, you actually believe that it is "made from sugar so it tastes like sugar" and all is good. But this is the real story: It's a synthetic chemical made by reacting sucrose (table sugar) with chlorine (the main ingredient in common household bleach). It was discovered by British-based agribusiness giant Tate & Lyle and researchers at a local university, who subsequently developed a partnership with McNeil Nutritionals, a subsidiary of Johnson & Johnson. Doesn't sound so home-sweet-home now, does it?

And while more than a hundred studies have been conducted to deem sucralose safe, and it is widely consumed by people in more than eighty countries worldwide, the CSPI cautions against its consumption. That lab in Italy that tested aspartame and published "flawed" studies indicating that it caused cancer in rats and mice looked at sucralose in 2012 and determined that it caused leukemia in mice that were exposed to it before birth. [15] You can take this information with a grain of "sugar," but if you are pregnant and suck in sucralose, please stop! And everyone else, tread lightly.

The author of *Artificial Sweeteners: Sugar-Free, But at What Cost,* an article published by Harvard Health Publications in 2012, quotes Dr. David Ludwig, an obesity and weight specialist at Boston Children's Hospital who has a great interest in any and all products developed to help people lose weight and keep weight off: "Non-nutritive sweeteners are far more potent than table sugar and high-fructose corn syrup. A minuscule amount produces a sweet taste comparable to that of sugar, without comparable calories. Overstimulation of sugar receptors from frequent use of these hyper-intense sweeteners may limit tolerance for more complex tastes." [16]

In other words, the author points out, "People who routinely use artificial sweeteners may start to find less intensely sweet foods, such as fruit, less appealing and unsweet foods, such as vegetables, downright unpalatable." [17]

So these sugar phonies could be doing more damage than you think. You have to decide for yourself what "safe" really means vis-a-vis your eats. There is plenty of info out there to poke holes in the case for the safety of artificial sweeteners.

NEOTAME (GRAS)

The folks who brought you aspartame (the NutraSweet Company, a division of the biochemical giant Monsanto) introduced chemical creation neotame, which was approved by the FDA and introduced to the U.S. market in 2002 and subsequently to the European Union in 2010.

While there have been one hundred corporate-sponsored studies supposedly proving neotame's safety, it is a sibling to aspartame. Basically, the NutraSweet Company took aspartame and added another chemical to the mix (3,3-dimethylbutyl), giving you neotame (and then sold their company and creation to private equity firm J.W. Childs).

Food manufacturers love neotame because it's really cheap, and very little of it has to be used since it is super sweet. Neotame is now widely used in processed foods though you won't find it in little packets at Starbucks just yet. Apparently the money guys behind it have big hopes and dreams for this New Age sweetener, according to their website: "Neotame, the culmination of over 20 years of research, is an exciting new sweetener and flavor enhancer that provides manufacturers flexibility in formulating great tasting products throughout their existing food and beverage portfolios. In addition, neotame's versatility provides for the development of entire new ranges of products that meet the ever-increasing demands of consumers. Neotame is the fastest-growing sweetener in the world and it is used in more than 1,000 products worldwide."[18]

And what, you may ask, are these products? Carbonated beverages like diet soda, juice drinks like Tampico, protein shakes, protein bars, and even pharmaceuticals. I wish I had more details here, but sadly neotame is somewhat undercover. The CSPI suggests that neotame is safe for consumption based on all *available* research. While I am all for an alternative to the overconsumption of sugar, I am not in any way an advocate for suspect additives. Who knows what will pop up about aspartame's snuggly sibling ten years from now? Bottom line: Who needs any touch of potential toxicity in their food?

On Other Sugar Substitutes

Sugar Alcohols (GRAS)

Most sugar alcohols are manufactured from cornstarch (and typically from genetically modified corn—see sidebar, "Genetic Modification Modified" on page 42 but also more on this in chapter 10). Their name is somewhat misleading as they are neither sugar nor alcohol, but their chemical structure resembles both. Just like the artificials, they are made in a lab.

Consumers love them because they serve up sweetness but are considered "safe" for diabetics (they don't cause a sudden increase in blood sugar because they are metabolized differently than the real stuff); have fewer calories than sugar; and don't promote tooth decay. And the food industry is over the moon because sugar alcohols also add texture to foods, retain moisture, prevent browning when heated, and, most important, allow companies to label their products as "sugar-free."

Since sugar-free is the way to be, Americans are consuming quite a bit of this stuff. Beware, because overconsumption of these substitutes (which happens all too often) can cause bloating and diarrhea. And while sugar alcohols don't cause a *sudden* increase in blood sugar, they still cause an increase. So caution against the various types of sugar alcohols: erythritol, hydrogenated starch hydrolysates, isomalt, lactitol, maltitol, mannitol, sorbitol, and xylitol.

Novel Sweeteners (GRAS Excluding Whole-Leaf and Crude Stevia Extracts)

The quest for sweetness without the calories and blood sugar effect continues, and you will find some up-and-comers in a new category of sugar substitutes that defines itself as "various types of sweeteners from multiple sources." Included in the novel category are stevia (as well PureVia by Pepsi and Truvia by Coke), fructo-oligosaccharide (FOS), tagatose, and trehalose.

While whole-leaf stevia and crude stevia extracts are not approved for use by the FDA, highly refined stevia is generally recognized as safe. The compound that makes stevia sweet (Reb A) is extracted from the leaf itself through a brewing and purification process, and in the Pepsi and Coke versions, it is combined with other ingredients like sugar alcohols and natural flavors to make a "natural" zero-calorie sweetener. Industry and consumers love this stuff and use it liberally despite studies in the 1980s that linked it to reproductive problems and cancer in animals, in addition to a 2008 report out of UCLA emphasizing the need for more testing (and not from the companies who are making the stuff), because of evidence that derivatives of stevia damage DNA.[19]

According to the Sugar Association, other novel sweeteners to keep an eye out for are FOS, tagatose (also known as Naturlose), and trehalose. FOS comes from a starch called inulin that is found in many plants; tagatose occurs naturally in dairy products, so for commercial use it is manufactured from lactose (milk sugar) through a patented process; and trehalose is a sugar inherently found in everything from honey to lobster, but it is manufactured from cornstarch for commercial use. The FDA granted GRAS status to all of these novel sweeteners, and they are permeating the food supply to add sweetness to your sweets. While there is no cause for concern at this time, and each novel sweetener comes from plants (or animals), they do go through a manufacturing process that takes the sweetening compound out of its natural environment, thus altering it from its natural form. This in and of itself is concerning to me.

Uncategorized Sweeteners (Undetermined)

Somewhat hot off the press is advantame by Ajinomoto. According to the company's website, Advantame is an innovative new ingredient derived from aspartame (the highly controversial artificial sweetener) and vanillin (fake vanilla flavor). It's an artificial sweetener and flavor in one that can be used to enhance existing flavors in foods and confections. You need a very little bit to go a long way (so low use), and it's cheap. Oh, and it can also mask the off-taste of the somewhat unsavory Reb-A, Splenda, and acesulfame K.

It is apparently safe, and right now, it's being used overseas. But it is still under scrutiny by the FDA for GRAS status.

Genetic Modification Modified

While chapter 10 is entirely devoted to the topic of genetically modified organisms (GMOs), also referred to as genetic engineering, let me offer a brief explanation now so you can begin to understand a serious issue that is facing your food supply and likely your health.

GMOs are plants or animals created through gene-splicing techniques (also called biotechnology). This technology merges DNA from different species, creating potentially unstable combinations of plant, animal, bacterial, and viral genes that cannot occur in nature (or in traditional cross-breeding). Almost all commercial GMOs are engineered mainly to tolerate direct application of herbicides and/or to produce an insecticide. Monsanto (one of the leading biotech companies behind GMOs) claims that the world needs genetic modification (more on this later). But truth be told, many notable scientists, health experts, and food-industry watchdogs have been questioning GMOs' safety since they were introduced to market twenty-plus years ago. My take: you have been a lab rat in one of the greatest science experiments of all time, thanks to biotech. But hopefully *What the Fork* will help you understand the issues, so you can decide if you want to go for the GMOs or fight for your right to know, meaning truth in labeling.

The Better for You Alternatives

I urge you to avoid artificial sweeteners at all costs, and I hope you are convinced that there is enough evidence to question their safety as a whole, whether from a scientific point of view or a commonsense perspective. While I don't advocate for sugar alcohols or novel sweeteners, they are a better option if consumed in moderation. Ideally, though, I prefer that you eat the real deal.

For those of you who need to mind your blood sugar, turn to the idea of food combining—meaning that if you are going to consume something with sugar, make sure you do so with some fat or protein, as that will slow down sugar metabolism. For example, ditch the sugar-free, fat-free yogurt for the real stuff—plain yogurt with a spot of honey, maple syrup, or even some real-deal fruit jam topped with a small portion of nuts—a more wholesome and healthy choice.

CHAPTER 5

Sugar and Its Many Euphemisms*

My husband is like most Americans. Married to me or not, he is a product of his upbringing and the food industry's target marketing. In fact, one day when we were in Whole Foods, he picked up the organic version of Cocoa Krispies and attempted to put it in the cart. I took one look at the box, then at him, and just shook my head.

"What?" he said. "It's organic!"

I responded with, "Just 'cause it's organic and at Whole Foods *does not* mean that it is healthy."

There is not a highly processed sugared cereal that I would consider healthy. Oftentimes, sugar is listed at least two times, if not more, in the ingredient list. But while his version lists it twice as "organic evaporated cane juice" and again as "organic molasses," the conventional counterpart lists it four times as "sugar," "semisweet chocolate" (that includes "sugar" and "dextrose") and "malt flavoring." So would I recommend that you buy the organic version instead of the original? Only if these crispy bursts of chocolate are a Can't Live Without item (more on this in Section Two). If not, how about ditching the crunch, 'cause any way you bite it, both cereals are laced with unnecessary sugar.

Did you know that there are roughly fifty different ways that sugar can be listed on your ingredient labels, so that getting duped into buying a

---

*No FDA regulations apply as sugar (and most of its derivatives) are food versus food additives (whether requiring premarket approval or GRAS).

high-sugar product is highly likely? Check this out: agave, Barbados sugar, barley malt, beet sugar, brown sugar, buttered syrup, cane juice crystals, cane sugar, caramel, carob syrup, castor sugar, confectioners' sugar, corn syrup, corn syrup solids, date sugar, demerara sugar, dextrin, dextrose, diastatic malt, diatase, Florida crystals, fructose, fruit juice, fruit juice concentrate, galactose, glucose, glucose solids, golden sugar, golden syrup, grape sugar, high-fructose corn syrup, honey, icing sugar, invert sugar, lactose, maltodextrin, malt syrup, maple syrup, molasses, muscovado sugar, panela, raw sugar, refiner's syrup, rice syrup, sorghum syrup, Sucanat, sucrose, sugar, treacle, turbinado sugar, and yellow sugar.

There is little point in defining all of them (they are largely equal when it comes to your consumption and the end result), but the advice is the same: Don't get fooled by sugar and its many euphemisms—clearly the sweet stuff can rear its head in varied ways in your food.

Briefly on Organic

According to the USDA National Organic Program (NOP), "organic is a labeling term indicating that a food or other agricultural product integrates cultural, biological, and mechanical practices that foster cycling of resources, promotes ecological balance, and conserves biodiversity. Synthetic fertilizers, sewage sludge, irradiation, and genetic engineering are not permitted." For plants, the organic seal "verifies that irradiation, sewage sludge, synthetic fertilizers, prohibited pesticides [certain NOP approved chemicals are allowed to be used in organic farming and processing], and genetically modified organisms were not used." As for animals, it "verifies that producers met animal health and welfare standards, did not use antibiotics or growth hormones, used 100% organic feed, and provided animals with access to the outdoors."[1]

What They Are

"Sugar" is the generalized term for sweet-flavored substances that typically derive from processed sugarcane or sugar beets (corn is another sugar "starter," but more on that later).

To simplify a rather complex process, I will just say that freshly harvested sugarcane goes straight to a sugar mill, where it is pressed to separate the cane from the juice. The liquid is then boiled to eliminate moisture, resulting in a thick syrup with some crystallization—this is *real* raw sugar, impurities and all. Then it goes from the mill to the refinery, where the sweet stuff goes through another process called carbonatation and additional filtration to remove the roughly 2 percent impurities (including the iron and calcium-rich molasses, a by-product of sugar processing) from the raw sugar. Once these impurities are removed, the liquid still has color, so it is passed through carbon filters or, in some instances, bovine bone char (yup, crushed-up pieces of bones from a cow) to remove the color. So, technically your sugar is not "bleached," as no whitening chemical such as chlorine is used to get the color out. The result is an unpigmented liquid that moves into pans for more boiling and highly specific refining into the many sugars that you see on supermarket shelves today.

Unlike sugarcane, sugar beets don't go from mill to refinery; they are processed under one roof. Once harvested, they are sliced into French fry–like shapes before going through a diffuser to extract the sugar molecule into a water solution. The liquid is then filtered to remove the impurities (including an inedible form of molasses). Once the impurities are gone, the beet sugar goes through the same whitening process as sugarcane and is then further refined into many forms.

According to the Sugar Association (the result of a merger between the U.S. Cane Sugar Refining Association and the U.S. Beet Sugar Association), there are three categories of the sweet stuff (whether from cane or beets):

WHITE SUGAR

Basically, the white stuff is anything that is granulated to a fine or extra-fine sugar, so essentially it's the most refined form of sugar. You can find it in every eatery, whether granulated, in cubes, or in packets; in that bag or box at the grocery store; and in many processed foods on the market.

BROWN SUGAR

While still refined, some of the molasses is left in (in varying quantities in each type). You can find turbinado sugar (aka sugar in the raw) in the same places where you find white sugar. Evaporated cane juice (such as Sucanat), the common light and dark brown sugar*, muscovado or Barbados sugar (a British specialty with a strong molasses flavor), and demerara sugar (also popular in England) are all your run-of-the-mill browns.

LIQUID SUGAR

Liquid sugar is basically sugar syrup (or simple syrup), meaning that white sugar is dissolved in water (typically 1 part sugar to 1 part water). Invert sugar is another option whereby the liquid sugar is treated with an acid to "invert" it, making a more concentrated sugar that won't recrystallize if liquid is boiled off, so it is ideal for retaining moisture in processed foods.

Now on to corn—I surely can't leave it behind, as there is plenty of sugar on the market that comes from the yellow, including the controversial corn syrup and high-fructose corn syrup (HFCS), as well as caramel, dextrin, dextrose, fructose, glucose syrup, golden syrup, and maltodextrin, to name a few.

When corn (commonly genetically modified) is processed into edibles such as cornmeal, corn flour, corn oil, or maltodextrin, there are natural

---

*Brown sugar can come from sugarcane, like the common Domino's brand as well as sugar beets. If the latter, it is "painted" with molasses from sugarcane (because the molasses from sugar beets is inedible) like the Pioneer and Big Chief brands brought to you by the Michigan Sugar Company. You will never know the real source of your sugar unless the package says "pure cane sugar."

starchy by-products of manufacturing. It is these leftovers that get the corn syrup makeover. They travel through an extraction process that begins by introducing enzymes to this grain (fresh corn is considered a vegetable, but dried corn is considered a grain) to break the starch down into sugar. More enzymes are added, and then acids to facilitate the conversion of the starch to sugar, and then voilà, corn syrup and HFCS is born.

The Corn Syrup Conundrum

The Corn Refiners Association and the Sugar Association are in a constant battle. Many years after the corn syrup community pushed themselves into the food processing industry, trying to replace sugar (from cane and beets) with cheaper sweets, HFCS is finally losing market share to seemingly healthier counterparts like real sugar and its many euphemisms (as well as the artificials).

As a result, Big Corn decided to ask the FDA to rename HFCS to "corn sugar," and lo and behold, the request was denied. Apparently the FDA defines sugar as a solid, dried, and crystallized food—not syrup.

So, while the battle between Big Corn and Big Sugar continues, it may all be for naught as a growing body of research suggests that HFCS, and its too-close-for-comfort relative, sugar, may contribute to diseases that kill hundreds of thousands of Americans every year. In fact, according to research conducted by the Harvard School of Public Health, "roughly 180,000 obesity-related deaths worldwide are associated with the consumption of sugary drinks. The abstract, presented at an American Heart Association scientific conference in New Orleans, linked drinking sugar-sweetened beverages to 133,000 diabetes deaths, 44,000 deaths from cardiovascular diseases, and 6,000 cancer deaths. The researchers found that 78% of these deaths were in low- and middle-income countries."[2]

So if you dial down your total consumption of added sugars, you could surely reduce the risk of chronic disease and possible death.

While I consider sugarcane, sugar beets, and corn the top three "sugar starters," the sweet stuff can also come from other plants such as rice (rice syrup), barley (barley malt), cactus (agave), the maple tree (maple syrup), and various fruits (or fruit juice and fruit juice concentrate), including the coconut. It can also come from bees (honey). All sugar initiators go through some form of processing (some less than others, with honey and maple syrup among the least processed), but in the end, it's all sugar.

Now that you have the 411, I have to go a little "science geek" on you. Most sugars, as you know them, are sucrose—a combination of glucose and fructose. Carbohydrates (essentially anything from a plant) break down into single sugar molecules that are then absorbed directly into your bloodstream to help make your motor run. The most common molecules include glucose, dextrose (a type of glucose typically derived from cornstarch), fructose, and galactose.

Everything sugar has some combination of glucose and fructose, but the industry (including Big Corn and Big Sugar) spends a lot of money and time defending their sweets, and scientists debate over these mini-molecules. For instance, fructose is the belly fat culprit. But in the end this topic is being micromanaged to madness, and all you need to focus on is reducing your overall sugar intake because whether from sugarcane, sugar beets, corn, or any other source, it is still sugar.

Why They Are "Bad"

I am sure that you have more than an inkling as to why too much sugar is bad. And I am not talking fresh fruit, but the added sweet stuff (for those of you who may be wondering). According to "The Toxic Truth about Sugar," published in 2012 in the prestigious journal *Nature*, researchers concluded that HFCS and sugar (any kind) are as addictive as cigarettes and alcohol, and that overconsumption of both is the driving force behind the worldwide epidemics of obesity and type 2 diabetes (the type associated with obesity). An estimated $150 billion a year is the price tag for sugar-related diseases in America alone.[3]

While I am not going to vilify HFCS, as it is clear that this highly processed sugar has some partners in crime, I must admit that I am not a fan of "corn sugar" for two simple reasons: (1) It is highly processed compared to real sugar and (2) in 2011, 88 percent of the U.S. corn crop was genetically modified.[4] And most likely that percentage has expanded since.

On sugar beets, the Non-GMO Project, an NGO devoted to preserving and building sources of non-GMO products, educating consumers, and providing verified non-GMO choices, found that in 2010, approximately 95 percent of the U.S. sugar beet crop was genetically modified. Evidently, a large percentage of anything sweet can be chock-full of GMOs.

So aim to understand where your sugar comes from and manage your overall intake no matter what the source. And just to make me happy, how about keeping the sugar you *must* consume as pure as possible?

The Better for You Alternatives

Speaking of pure, my go-to sweetener is honey because it is the least processed of all sweeteners. However, my true love is maple syrup (not the fake stuff made with corn syrup and artificial maple flavoring) and brown rice syrup, despite the fact that both are processed through extraction, the addition of enzymes in some cases and heating.

So very simply, whatever your sugar of choice is, try to consume *less* (even if you switch to honey). The American Heart Association suggests that men limit *added* sugar to 36 grams (9 teaspoons) per day, and women to 24 grams (6 teaspoons) per day. Again, I am not talking about sugar in fruit or other carbohydrates, but rather the sugar that is oh-so-generously added to almost everything processed. To translate, one bottle of a popular sports drink has roughly 32.5 grams of sugar.

Thus, your first line of attack is to limit your intake of sugary beverages and processed foods, as these packaged prizes are loaded with sugar.

Everything from soups and sauces to alternative milks (like soy milk) and yogurt contain sinful amounts of sweetness. Now that you know the many faces of sugar, avoid products with unnecessary additions (there are plenty on the market without the added sweet). Reclaim control over what goes in your body.

CHAPTER 6

Trans Fats (Hydrogenated Oils)*

Do you remember the days of margarine? Fabio, his flowing hair, and I Can't Believe It's Not Butter!®? I call this food history moment the "Margarine Chronicles." Basically, this bright yellow, butterlike substance was the food industry's response to growing concern over saturated fat (the "bad for you" fat found in butter and other animal products) and its role in heart disease.

Rewind to the late 1850s. German pathologist Rudolf Virchow posited that the accumulation of lipids (saturated fat and cholesterol) in the blood caused the hardening of arteries (atherosclerosis), and thus heart disease. His theory was dubbed the *lipid hypothesis*.

As the prevalence of atherosclerosis skyrocketed in the mid-twentieth century, so did the number of scientific studies aiming to find a cause. The most notable studies to date are the Framingham Heart Study, the Multiple Risk Factor Intervention Trial, and the Lipid Research Clinics Coronary Primary Prevention Trial, all funded by a division of the National Institute of Health. Their conclusion so far is that this lipid hypothesis may not be all that it's cracked up to be. There are many other supposed factors, including trans fat intake and overconsumption of sugar, that contribute to heart disease.

---

*Currently Generally Recognized as Safe (GRAS) but will soon be deemed a food additive requiring pre-market approval by the FDA.

What They Are

All hydrogenated oils (aka partially hydrogenated oils) are made by taking vegetable oil (the unsaturated, good-for-you fat), whether from cottonseed, canola, or soy (some of the top genetically modified contenders), and pumping hydrogen into the liquid under high pressure to make it solid at room temperature. My favorite example is Crisco, the very first hydrogenated oil product made from cottonseed oil, which was introduced to market by Procter and Gamble in 1911. Why? To offer a cheaper alternative to animal fats such as lard and butter.

The guy who created hydrogenation in the late 1800s was French chemist Paul Sabatier. Then in 1901, Wilhelm Normann, an award-winning German chemist, took Sabatier's discovery and applied it to fats, creating what we now know as trans fats. Or, as I like to call them, man-made fats. Both were award-winning scientists. I applaud advancements in science— they are both incredible and valuable—but I find it increasingly astonishing that the folks who create chemicals or chemical processes to make your food more desirable rather than healthy receive such accolades for their discoveries (think back to the woman who received the "award" for extracting vanilla flavor from cow poop).

While margarine, first called oleomargarine, was around in the 1800s (prior to Crisco), it was made from beef fat and offered a satisfying and less expensive alternative to butter for the armed forces and the lower classes. As World War II came with a shortage of butter and subsequent rationing, oleomargarine gained a following. And it hasn't lost popularity since— essentially it looks like butter and tastes like butter, but *is not* butter.

Margarine has gone through many iterations since the 1930s. It began with beef fat, then shifted to hydrogenated vegetable oils around the 1950s, when the American Heart Association stated that reducing saturated fats like lard and butter can reduce your chance of getting heart disease (back to the lipid hypothesis). So today, a percentage of margarine in the marketplace is some combination of hydrogenated oils, water, whey (the liquid by-product of cheese production), milk, chemical preservatives, and artificial colors and flavors (though some nonhydrogenated versions are available, even more purist ones, as noted at the end of this chapter). Unilever, the company that brings you everything from Dove and Vaseline to Hellman's and Lipton, is one of the leading global innovators and manufacturers of margarine under the most recognized brand names, such as Brummel & Brown, Country Crock, Flora, Imperial, Promise, and I Can't Believe It's Not Butter!*

But it's not all about Crisco and margarine. Hydrogenated oils, in one form or another, have been used in the manufacturing of food products for decades. The conversion of liquid oils into solid (hydrogenated) or semi-solid (partially hydrogenated) fats is favored by the food industry because they are cheap (of course) and more stable and have a longer shelf life than their animal fat counterparts like butter. Also, hydrogenation allows the industry to manipulate the oil to a consistency that is perfect for spreads, frying (whether for the fast-food industry or common snack foods like chips) or commercial baked goods like breads, bread crumbs, crackers, cookies, and cakes.

Why They Are "Bad"

In the 1950s, the American Heart Association told you to reduce your consumption of saturated fats. Too much could lead to heart disease. The food industry's response was hydrogenated vegetable oils, whether in the form of Crisco or spreads like margarine, which were replacements for lard and butter in many processed foods. Health advocates even lobbied the fast-food industry to stop frying in beef tallow and switch to the "healthier" hydrogenated oil.

Even *I* bought into the "Margarine Chronicles," consuming enough soy margarine to choke a horse in the early 1990s. That was the pseudovegan stage of my life, so margarine was the solution for a spread on my daily grainy toast. At my annual physical, my doctor told me that my cholesterol had skyrocketed *even though I was a vegan.* That made no sense whatsoever, as there was really nothing in my diet that could promote high cholesterol (such as saturated fat). My basic instinct told me to remove the margarine, and sure enough, a month later my cholesterol was perfect.

Right around the same time, many research studies were conducted linking trans fat consumption with elevated LDL (bad) cholesterol. Most notably, *The Lancet* published an article by Walter Willet and his team at Harvard University concluding that the consumption of partially hydrogenated vegetable oils may contribute to the occurrence of heart disease.[1]

Finally there was enough evidence to get the government to do something. As of January 1, 2006 (a freakin' thirteen years after this study was published), trans fats became an official fat category on all Nutrition Facts labels, meaning that all food makers were required to list the quantity of these man-made and potentially lethal fats alongside the saturated fat and unsaturated fat content. This translated into many industry giants reformulating their foods with healthier fats. Even Crisco has a trans fat–free option.

But there is a catch here. While trans fats are now labeled in italics on Nutrition Facts panels, according to the FDA, a food can claim it is trans fat–free while still containing up to half a gram (0.5 g) of hydrogenated oils. So be sure to check ingredient lists for "hydrogenated oil" or "partially hydrogenated oil," as the Nutrition Facts can fib but the ingredient lists (even if less than 0.5 g) cannot.

The FDA Trans Fats Update

In early November 2013, the FDA issued a Federal Register Notice stating the following:

"Based on new scientific evidence and the findings of expert scientific panels, the Food and Drug Administration has tentatively determined that partially hydrogenated oils (PHOs) . . . are not generally recognized as safe (GRAS) for any use in food based on current scientific evidence establishing the health risks associated with the consumption of trans fat, and therefore that PHOs are food additives. . . . If finalized, this would mean that food manufacturers would no longer be permitted to sell PHOs, either directly or as ingredients in another food product, without prior FDA approval for use as a food additive."[2]

Remember, it was more than twenty years ago that *The Lancet* published the study vilifying trans fats. Sadly the researchers' concerns fell on deaf ears, and you have suffered as a result. When will the food industry and government *stop* playing roulette with your health? I wish I had an answer. As of now, this notice has not been finalized, meaning that there is no set date for the mandatory removal of trans fats from foods without prior FDA approval. According to the agency, they are "soliciting comments on how such an action would impact small businesses and how to ensure a smooth transition if a final determination is issued."[3]

But do know this: When the trigger is pulled, food manufacturers will likely replace trans fats with palm oil (made from the fruit of the palm oil tree); palm kernal oil (made from the seed); and perhaps coconut oil, all high in saturated fats. Although these oils are healthier than trans fats, high intake could be a risk factor for heart disease, so be wary of overconsumption. Concern doesn't end there, however; according to the Rainforest Alliance, the international nongovernmental organization that works to conserve biodiversity and ensure sustainable livelihood, "We share the concerns of many about the impact of expanding oil palm plantations on the rainforests, particularly in the Southeast Asia region and especially on the islands of Borneo and Sumatra. Deforestation in this region, as in the Amazon, is one of the most urgent challenges facing environmentalists today."[4]

As I see it, the goal here is to solve one problem (overconsumption of trans fats, leading to disease), not to cause another (further environmental destruction and overconsumption of too much saturated fat in the form of palm oil). Clearly, your food choice not only makes a difference in your health, but is also part of a much bigger picture—one I encourage you to start thinking about if you haven't already.

The Better for You Alternatives

Since the implementation of the new labeling laws, the food industry has shifted greatly as consumers have grown concerned about trans fat intake. While Crisco and margarine are still stocked on most grocery store shelves, they both have trans fat–free options. But don't forget to read the ingredient lists, as they often are packed with other Top-Rated Terminators like chemical preservatives and artificial flavors and colors. Though more purist options like trans fat–free shortening by Spectrum and Earth Balance spread do exist, keep in mind that most are highly processed and contain fillers and "natural" flavors.

As far as your snacks and sweets go, choose ones that are *truly* void of man-made fats. Remember, the Nutrition Facts can fib, so always aim to read the ingredient lists to ensure that the ubiquitous "hydrogenated oils" or "partially hydrogenated oils" are really MIA. Some of the biggest culprits are cookies, cakes, crackers, chips, canned soups, and bread crumbs. So if these products boast "trans fat–free," definitely do a double take.

When it comes to fast food, if ya gotta do it, I imagine that avoiding trans fats is not a priority for you. But to make me happy, how about asking if the company cooks with hydrogenated oils and for what items? And if your choice is doused in man-made grease, pick another menu option. Even small changes can make a big difference.

The bottom line is that I would like you to kiss Fabio good-bye and eat butter, not shortening or margarine (even if touted as trans fat–free) because these buckets of brew are highly processed. I would like you to avoid all products containing any amount of trans fat (the research proves that they are unnatural-born killers). If you need to make that perfect piecrust, a little butter or some coconut oil won't hurt. If you have issues with dairy, drizzle a little extra virgin olive oil on your bread. Or if you absolutely need that buttery flavor, opt for a better-for-you brand like Earth Balance.

CHAPTER 7

Pesticides*

Paul Francois is a forty-something grain farmer living in southeast France. Like many farmers, he uses pesticides to manage his crop. These chemicals kill everything from weeds to insects, while ensuring that the plants grow and are good for eating. In 2004, after applying (and accidentally inhaling) the chemical weed killer Lasso, made by Monsanto (the biotech giant that also created saccharin and is one of the leading innovators of genetic modification), Francois didn't feel too fabulous. He began experiencing neurological problems, including memory loss, headaches, and stammering. As a result, Francois went for the jugular and sued Monsanto, blaming them for not providing adequate warnings on their product label. Amazingly, Francois won; in February 2012, Monsanto was found culpable of chemical poisoning. It was the *first time* a pesticide maker was found guilty of such a crime.

The idea of getting sick after inhaling any chemical is plausible. But you would hope that it wasn't one that is also being used on your food. The Lasso incident definitely raised *my* eyebrows. Although you won't take in the amount that Mr. Francois did in one fell swoop, you do consume plenty over time if you ingest nonorganic plant foods (like most Americans).

In 1991, the USDA initiated the Pesticide Data Program (PDP) to test commodities (any large-scale crop [or animal food] including fruits and vegetables, grains, beans, and sugar that is grown and sold for processing

*Environmental Protection Agency sets tolerances of chemicals; FDA enforces tolerance levels.

and/or packaging, then resale) for pesticide residues. The USDA teams up with the Environmental Protection Agency to determine what foods they are going to test on a yearly basis. But wait, shouldn't all foods be tested? The EPA had this to offer in 2012:

> The newest data from the PDP program confirms that pesticide residues in food do not pose a safety concern for Americans. EPA remains committed to a rigorous, science-based, and transparent regulatory program for pesticides that continues to protect people's health and the environment.[1]

With the PDP now in place, the Environmental Working Group (EWG), one of the nation's preeminent environmental health research and advocacy organizations devoted to protecting human health and the environment, had extensive data on which to build one of their highly credible consumer tools—Shopper's Guide to Pesticides in Produce™, also known as the Dirty Dozen Plus™ and the Clean 15™ (available online and as a smartphone app). In 2012, the EWG had this to say:

- The highest pesticide residue levels are found on apples, strawberries, grapes, peaches, and imported nectarines.
- The most contaminated vegetables are celery, spinach, sweet bell peppers, cucumbers, potatoes, cherry tomatoes, and hot peppers.
- Every sample of imported nectarines tested positive for pesticides; 99 percent of apple samples tested positive for at least one pesticide residue.
- The average potato had a much higher total weight of pesticides than any other food crop.
- A single grape tested positive for fifteen pesticides. The same was true for a single sweet bell pepper. Single samples of celery, cherry tomatoes, and sweet bell peppers tested positive for thirteen different pesticides apiece.[2]

So even though your food is loaded with residues of toxic chemicals (at subtoxic levels) as noted by the EWG, and you are exposed to low doses of these compounds over a long period of time, your government claims your eats are still safe for consumption. And perhaps they are, but at what cost?

What They Are

Pesticides are chemicals used to kill anything unsavory that wants to destroy your food while it's growing. According to the National Pesticide Information Center (NPIC)—a cooperative between Oregon State University and the EPA to provide objective, science-based information about pesticides and pesticide-related topics that enable people to make informed decisions about these chemicals and their use—the following categories of pesticides are used on food: insecticides, rodenticides, herbicides, and fungicides. The EPA notes that these chemicals are used on edibles to prevent, destroy, repel, or mitigate "pests" including insects, mice, and other animals; unwanted plants (like weeds); and fungi and microorganisms (like bacteria and viruses). And a whopping 5.1 billion pounds of pesticides are used each year to keep your crops cropping.

Pursuant to the NPIC, these chemical concoctions contain both active ingredients and other ingredients. The actives are used to kill, control, or repel the "pest." And the others may do a variety of jobs, like spreading the active ingredients around and/or reducing unnecessary drift.

While thousands of chemicals are used to create these plant and animal killers, a small handful of them can be grouped according to their effects on the "pests." For example, organophosphates *irreversibly* inactivate the enzyme effective for nerve function (think nerve gas) in insects—as well as in humans and many other animals, I might add (but apparently not enough to cause harm). Their close relative, carbamates, have the same function, but the damage is reversible. Organochlorines like DDT that were once commonly used in agriculture have been "banned" due to their *persistent* health and environmental effects, but they were still being used as recently as 2012, according to the EWG. Thankfully, the EPA and chemical companies have finally agreed to terminate the use of organochlorines on your food in the United States, but they are still being used abroad (though thankfully *not* being imported to the United States). Regardless, these compounds linger in the environment, so don't be surprised if they still show up on your food for quite some time.

Pursuant to standards set by the EPA, chemical manufacturers (like Bayer, DuPont, Dow, Monsanto, and Syngenta) evaluate their very own creations for specific toxicities (like carcinogenicity and neurotoxicity). *Let me repeat, the people who make the chemicals are in charge of testing them for use on your food.* And, once the *i*'s are dotted and *t*'s are crossed, the data gets submitted to the EPA for review, approval, and specific use determination.

Based on the data submitted, the EPA determines if the chemical is deemed safe for your eats through a lengthy process of risk assessment and risk management. Despite the fact that the chemical can cause cancer or neurological problems at high doses, the EPA determines the lowest dose that produces effects, then knocks that down one hundred to one thousand times depending on the data to determine an acceptable level that is *expected* to cause *no harm*. Then, other considerations are taken into account including possible exposure from drinking water and the environment. Finally, the EPA sets pesticide residue tolerances—the amount of pesticide residue that can remain in or on each treated food making it "safe" for consumption.

Multiple nongovernmental organizations like the Environmental Working Group, Food and Water Watch (a rock-star consumer rights group focused on corporate and government accountability relating to food, water, and fishing), and several other organizations listed in Appendix E, "Redeemable Resources," work day in and day out to expose the truth and nothing but the truth about your food and water, pushing government to do the right thing. Tune into who they are and what they do and be grateful that *your health and the health of the environment (and all the gifts it has to offer)* are truly their bottom line.

Why They Are "Bad"

Back to Paul Francois. Pesticides are toxic chemicals and, if consumed in large quantities, can lead to serious health problems—that's why the Environmental Protection Agency is so deeply involved. While the EPA sets pesticide limits that are safe for consumption, I would be remiss to say that I do not have some serious concerns about these chemicals.

For one thing, just because pesticides are used on plants doesn't mean that they stay on plants. Pesticides are most commonly applied through mechanical sprayers, especially in conventional agriculture. Although great precautions are supposed to be taken, chemical particles travel through the air, get absorbed into the soil, and run off into your water, making for some serious pesticide porridge in your environment (and that of other living creatures around you—even ones that you consume). Thus, problems with pesticides are not limited to your plant food.

In 1993, the National Academy of Sciences, another NGO "charged with providing independent, objective advice to the nation on matters related to science and technology," issued the report *Pesticides in the Diets of Infants and Children*. And here are the highlights: Even though pesticide application has improved crop yield, increasing the quantity of available fresh fruits and vegetables, pesticides may also cause harm, damaging the environment and accumulating in ecosystems. Depending on dose, some pesticides can cause a range of adverse effects on human health, including cancer, acute and chronic injury to the nervous system, lung damage, reproductive dysfunction, and possibly dysfunction of the endocrine and immune systems. The safety of pesticides has primarily been tested on "sexually mature animals," but not on infants, children, the elderly, or those with health conditions; thinner skin, added fat, and compromised organ systems make it difficult for the body to extricate these chemicals. Thus the current regulatory system considers only the average exposure of the entire population.[3]

So thank your lucky stars that NGOs exist to raise the red flag on decisions that the government is or *is not* making to protect you from profit powerhouses who want to make your food "healthier." The EWG has a no-holds-barred approach to keeping the consumer informed about pesticide residues on fruits and vegetables. And according to this food watchdog, quite shamefully there is plenty to balk at with respect to baby food.

Of almost six hundred samples each of green beans, pears, and sweet potatoes processed as baby food in 2011, the green beans tested positive for five pesticides, including the toxic organophosphates methamidophos and acephate[4] (remember, the ones that *irreversibly* affect nerve function). Although these chemicals can no longer be used in home gardens or for other forms of pest control (though they still do exist in a particular fly strip), they continue to be used in large-scale agricultural operations (the organochlorines are the banned ones). In other words, you will still find residues on your food.

Pears that were processed for baby food had eleven pesticides. Iprodi-one, categorized by the EPA as a probable human carcinogen, was detected in several samples. But there is more—iprodione is not registered with the EPA for use on pears, so its presence in this baby food was a violation of FDA regulations (the agency responsible for enforcing tolerances set by the EPA). As far as the sweet potatoes go, they were squeaky clean.

In 2012, a report was published in *Endocrine Reviews* by a group of researchers at Tufts University noting that low-dose, long-term exposure to endocrine-disrupting chemicals such as those found in many pesticides have adverse effects on overall human health, "including links to infertility, cardiovascular disease, obesity, cancer and other disorders."[5] And although most of the studies reviewed in the report centered on individuals exposed through occupation or accidental subjection to high doses of environmental chemicals (like farmer Francois), these recent studies point to a broad range of issues facing the general population. Humans are not exposed to single chemicals but to mixtures of multiple chemicals. And very little is known about how these compounded chemicals act and react together. Thus, at this point, their effects on your health are, at best, uncharted territory.

While the U.S. government is working to limit the toxicity of pesticides, as well as exposure, they can't move fast enough. In the September 2012 issue of the *Annals of Internal Medicine*, Stanford University researchers concluded that people who eat organic significantly reduce pesticide concentrations in their bodies.[6] So while you may not be able to rely on the government to keep you safe from food, you can learn how to navigate the food options available. And honestly, who wouldn't want to reduce unwelcome chemical levels in their body?

The Better for You Alternatives

If you are anything like me, you can't buy organic 100 percent of the time because of the high cost, so I like to navigate fruits and vegetables with the help of EWG's Shopper's Guide to Pesticides in Produce™—more commonly known as the Dirty Dozen Plus™ and the Clean 15™. You can download the app onto your smartphone to give you the facts at your fingertips. Basically, this is my trusted tool to determine which foods I will always aim to buy organic, and which are okay to consume nonorganic. Whether or not produce is organic, I wash with wellness in mind. A good vegetable brush, some old-fashioned water, and a little scrub muscle do an okay job to remove the stuff on the outside. Oh, and for those of you who like those fancy vegetable sprays, there is no solid evidence showing that they are any better than water (so save your money).

But please bear in mind that eating plants with pesticides, in the end, is better than not eating any plants at all.

The Lowdown on Local
(Even If It's Not Organic)

I am all about supporting the local farmer—they are a dying breed thanks to industrialized agriculture. So in addition to keeping my food as clean as possible, I always try to buy within my community. The ideal is local organic (to eliminate any pesticide residues), but if I can't find it or it is too pricey, I will go local with chemicals. In the end, what I get from my friendly farmer is most likely fresher and more alive than the cross-continent counterpart.

Many townships, even booming cities, have *community-supported agriculture (CSA)*, in which you can buy a share in a farm and receive fresh produce weekly for several months throughout the year. Check out Local Harvest (localharvest.org) to find a CSA near you.

CHAPTER 8

Antibiotics*

Every summer, my family ventures to Maine for a week and we often visit friends on their beloved Bagaduce Family Farm. On the 120 acres of seaside pasture and woods, the handful of animals have plenty of legroom to rest, ruminate, and dine on the meadow. The pigs can root (dig with their snouts) for hours in the grassland or on the forest floor seeking subsurface yummies like bugs and worms, mushrooms and mosses. They also enjoy apples from the spotted orchard.

The cows, on the other hand, love their greens, constantly moving between blades of grass and perennial brush. They relish the many shrubs and trees adorning the acreage and nosh on everything from wild berries and apples to acorns. The poultry, whether chickens, ducks, geese, or guinea fowl, are truly free to roam, taking some level of ownership over any area they choose, whether the meadow or on the front stoop of the house. Their meal of choice, certified organic grain, is served to them around dinnertime. Isn't this the way animals raised for slaughter should live? For goodness' sake, they're giving their life to you for food, so as far as I am concerned, they should live it up while they can with some serious human help.

Bagaduce is bucolic and ideal. Factory farms are not. And according to GRACE Communications Foundation, the NGO that takes a close look at the environmental and public health effects of industrialized food systems, "Today, most farm animals in the United States are raised in con-

*FDA regulates as a drug for use in the food supply.

finement on huge industrialized systems that are more like factories than farms. These factory farms are large, profit driven companies which view animals as units of production rather than living creatures, and put efficiency and profits ahead of animal health and welfare."[1] And in turn, your health and welfare.

To give you a little visual, this is just some of what happens in concentrated animal feeding operations (CAFOs): The tails of dairy cows and pigs are cut, and egg-laying hens are debeaked to increase efficiency and safety (living quarters are very cramped, so who needs tails whipping and beaks pecking?); there is limited or no access to the outdoors; and conditions are unsanitary (lots and lots of feces). Are you sick to your stomach yet? Well, this is just the tip of the iceberg. Illness ensues as a result of undue stress and unsavory conditions. So your animals are dosed up on drugs. And guess what? An estimated 97 percent of all animal foods in the United States come from these stressed-out and sick creatures.

As sickness like pneumonia is all too common among animals that live (if you can call that living) in close quarters and unsanitary conditions, farmers often resort to giving their furry friends subtherapeutic levels of antibiotic medications in their daily munchies as a prophylactic measure—this apparently prevents the expected sickness and disease. So, thanks to Big Ag, the animals you eat essentially have no love and are addicted to drugs.

What They Are

Antibiotics are a group of potent medications used for fighting off bacterial infections. While bacteria are everywhere and even essential to some bodily functions, certain types can lead to illness. Surely you have taken antibiotics at some point in your life, for everything from skin to sinus to chest infections. While antibiotics are a necessary solution for treating many conditions in people and animals, they should not be fed daily to animals to ward off illness caused by unsanitary living conditions.

According to the Environmental Working Group, "Today, pharmaceuticals sold for use on food-producing animals amount to nearly 80% of the American antibiotics market."[2] A 2013 report from the Pew Charitable Trusts, an NGO working toward improving public policy, marked record high antibiotic sales for meat and poultry in 2011—Big Pharma sold 29.9 million pounds of drugs to Big Ag while only 7.7 million pounds went to treat sick humans.[3] Perhaps the following will offer some further insight into why your furry friends *need* the meds.

Dairy cattle live in either a tie-stall (picture a narrow parking space in a really large parking lot) with their necks tethered to a bar, a free-stall (picture the same parking space, except that the cows aren't tied and are free to roam and rest indoors on concrete floors), or a dry lot, an area without vegetation where animals hang out between scheduled milk production. Any way you slice it, cows are too close for comfort; they often suffer diseases of the feet due to standing for extended periods of time on concrete, or from hanging out in their own feces; and the mass production of milk often causes a painful udder disease. Undoubtedly, any or all of these situations can promote illness.

By the time the average American beef animal is around six months old, it has seen its last blade of grass. Cattle are ruminants, having the most highly evolved digestive organ on the planet, the rumen, which allows them to turn grass (a carbohydrate) into a protein. Cows are *meant* to eat grass, not corn, which is what they are fed from that six-month mark forward, after they enter their new digs—the feedlot. The reasoning behind corn is that it makes them grow faster and fatter (and it's the cheapest and easiest way to feed the animals). From a financial standpoint, this makes perfect sense to Big Ag, but from a human health standpoint, not so much. This *supersteer*, which subsists on a diet that it was not meant, by nature, to eat, takes eleven to fourteen months to grow to slaughter weight (rather than the healthy two-plus years for well-managed, grassfed, pasture-raised animals). So farmers see a lot of *feedlot bloat* (typically responsible for thousands of cattle deaths per year). In addition, liver abscesses and respiratory diseases are common. To prevent the outbreak of disease and to keep the animals alive and growing, farmers routinely give feedlot cattle subtherapeutic levels of meds in their daily diet. Giving drugs prophylactically continues to mask the failures of a truly broken system.

For good old Porky, the picture is even worse (if it can get any worse). Mamma pig (the sow) typically lives in confinement her entire life, most often confined within a narrow gestation stall (think of a super-narrow parking space where you can barely open your car door) with a slatted concrete floor. She can't even turn around. Once she pops out those piglets, their teeth and tails are clipped (farmers don't want the babes nibbling on each other's tails). The living conditions promote illness, including lung problems like pneumonia due to poor ventilation. So the farmers dose them up on drugs to make them "well." According to GRACE, the stress and mistreatment of pigs lead to illness and many piggy deaths before they ever get to the slaughterhouse.

While I am not going to cover all poultry, here is the general picture. Chickens raised for meat production are called broilers. So whether you eat a whole roast or parts alone, they all come from a broiler that is usually raised among thousands of others in a warehouselike structure with no access to the outdoors. Broilers are given growth-promoting antibiotics because farmers like to slaughter their birds in just over a month (compared to the three-plus months required for truly cared-for poultry). And as is all too common with factory farms, these birds are prone to illness due to the confinement and filth. So this means more drugs.

As far as hens (the chickens that lay your eggs) go, rarely are antibiotics given, since selling eggs with possible residues deems them unsellable. Conditions are pretty awful for most of our feathery friends—they are debeaked, kept in cages, and starved to prevent the natural molting process where birds shed and regrow feathers after laying eggs. As reported by GRACE, only 3.7 percent of the 281 million hens laying eggs in the United States are "cage-free." In other words, roughly 96 percent of hens spend their entire lives boxed in.[4]

According to the USDA, "[Cage-free] indicates that the flock was able to freely roam a building, room, or enclosed area with unlimited access to food and fresh water during their production cycle." But the reality is that these birds are often overcrowded and most don't have access to the outdoors. For "Free-Range/Free-Roaming," "producers must demonstrate to the Agency that poultry has been allowed access to the outside."[5] However, you will never really know where the poultry is roaming (dirt lot or pasture) and for how long. Both terms are neither regulated nor verified by a third party. More on these terms and many others in chapter 11.

Why They Are "Bad"

If your doctor suggested that you eat antibiotics with your food daily to prevent disease, would you do it? I highly doubt it. Long-term (even short-term) use of antibiotics comes with a cost. Excessive and prolonged use of these drugs tends to disrupt the happy balance of bacteria and yeast in your body and can lead to unrelenting illness. Animals are living creatures too, so antibiotics can disrupt their balance in a similar way.

Because of overuse of meds on animals, antibiotic-resistant bacteria have spawned in meat; in other words, the "bugs" can tolerate the drugs, so they don't get killed off. The prevalence of such bacteria as super-salmonella or campylobacter promotes food-borne illness and can trigger disease in ways never seen before. In 2013, the Environmental Working Group released the report *Superbugs Invade American Supermarkets*, in which they analyzed research and government tests of supermarket meats and concluded that disturbing amounts of the meat tested have incredibly high levels of antibiotic resistant bacteria. I hope you are sitting down—81 percent of ground turkey; 69 percent of pork chops; 55 percent of ground beef; and 39 percent of chicken breasts, wings, and thighs were found to be tainted with bacteria that could make you—and especially young children, pregnant women, the elderly, and people with weakened immune systems— super sick.[6] Folks, you are getting dosed up on potentially antibiotic-resistant bugs when you eat industrially farmed meat. In other words, if you get sick from the meat you eat, there's a good chance that the bug is resistant to drugs. According to the Centers for Disease Control and Prevention (CDC), "Each year in the United States, at least 2 million people become infected with bacteria that are resistant to antibiotics and at least 23,000 people die each year as a direct result of these infections."[7]

But there are ways you can minimize the risks and support farmers who are using antibiotics judiciously and appropriately.

The Better for You Alternatives

For anything animal, the ideal is buying products that bear the Animal Welfare Approved (AWA) or Certified Humane Raised and Handled (generally known as Certified Humane) seals of approval (more on this in chapter 11). Each boasts its own blue, green, and white label that dresses packages of meat, poultry, and eggs that have been certified (by a third party) according to the highest animal welfare and environmental standards, meaning the animals are treated humanely and drugs are used only when absolutely necessary (never routinely) for the health and welfare of individual animals. According to Animal Welfare Approved (AWA), the NGO that does the right thing, ensuring and verifying that animal products come from creatures raised with the highest animal welfare and environmental standards in mind, "[Our] program was founded in 2006 as a market-based solution to the growing consumer demand for meat, eggs and dairy products from animals treated with high welfare and managed with the environment in mind. You can trust in the AWA label while making food choices when you can't visit the farm yourself."[8]

Many organic brands hopefully support *truly* humane animal welfare practices and, as per National Organic Program (NOP) regulations, don't drug their animals in any way. However, according to Andrew Gunther, food and farming advocate and program director of AWA, "Although the simple antibiotic-free message may resonate with the public at large, the truth is that an all or nothing approach to antibiotic use in farming won't actually fix anything. In fact it is more likely to make things a whole lot worse."[9] The reality is that however well you look after animals, they can get sick—just as humans do. And when ill, they need medication to alleviate pain and suffering. So what happens to the meat from an animal in the organic program that is given drugs? Although it is perfectly safe to eat meat from animals that received antibiotics when they were sick (remember, animals in the organic program are not given subtherapeutic levels of any drugs), it can no longer be deemed USDA Organic and is removed from the program. Gunther adds, "When antibiotics are used appropriately to treat individual sickness, and where the correct withdrawal period is fully observed, there is no justification whatsoever to reject the meat, milk or eggs as second class."

Definitely go local if the farm is verified as noted; if it isn't verified, make sure you know the *right questions to ask* about how the animals were treated, fed, and drugged (you will get further guidance on this in sections two and three).

If humane treatment of animals is your thing (as it is mine), the only surefire way to confirm that your animals were looked after properly is to seek the AWA or Certified Humane seals of approval. You can find them in some mainstream markets; for example, the widely available Murray's poultry is Certified Humane. Also check out animalwelfareapproved.org and certifiedhumane.org to find a trusted farm to buy from. It may cost a little more, but your health is at stake. USDA Organic is also a good choice. Oh, and don't get fooled by label lingo like "cage-free," "pasture raised," or "grass fed." While the government defines these terms, none of them are truly regulated (more on this in chapter 11), so they could just be a bunch of empty promises. And, when dining out, don't be too shy to ask questions about the animals you are planning to order—you have a right to know where your food is coming from.

If you choose wisely when eating animals, it will surely make a difference in your health. You will be at little or no risk of consuming antibiotic-resistant bacteria and take in more omega-3 fatty acids (those highly anti-inflammatory and health-supportive fats) when you choose truly grassfed beef and pasture-raised poultry. Plus, you'll be helping the farmers who are *truly* doing the right thing and in turn the environment.

Something else to think about: How about reducing your fleshy consumption by subscribing to Meatless Monday (meatlessmonday.com)—a global movement with a very simple message: Once a week, cut the meat.

CHAPTER 9

Hormones*

I have never been much of a girly-girl. In fact, Barbie got a buzz cut and lived in the bowels of my closet. While cooking or pretending to be a nurse back in the 1970s was still stereotypically female, it didn't seem as bad to me as playing with dolls—I was a bit of a tomboy.

So in my tweens, when all the girls around me started to develop, I was completely unfazed—that is, until one unforgettable summer at my Adirondack camp, when my breasty bunkmates decided that it was cool to slap their hands on my still flat-as-a-board chest. And it was from that moment forward that every aspect of a girl's development became noticeable.

Consequently, telling you that girls today are maturing much earlier than they did thirty years ago is no lie. In fact, in 2010, *Pediatrics* published an article on puberty assessment in girls, noting that many girls are now developing breasts between the ages of seven and eight. That's four years younger than any tween.[1]

The exact reason why this is occurring is rather elusive, but several possible causes have been identified, including estrogen-like, hormone-disrupting chemicals used in plastics and the lining of cans packaging your food (see sidebar, "Boasting BPA-Free," page 201), as well as some of the pesticides pushed on your eats. There is another theory that perhaps the ever-present hormones given to anything that grazes (or is supposed to graze) to make them grow big and fast is prompting early puberty and possibly other ill effects.

---

*FDA regulates as a drug for use in the food supply.

What They Are

As agriculture began to industrialize in the early 1900s, farms became larger; the small, diverse farms that had produced everything from tomatoes to turkeys were no longer considered efficient. Thus farmsteads became specialized, ultimately driving the small guy out of town. As a result, market control was handed over to a handful of very powerful corporations.

To this day, the primary goal of Big Ag is to profit—meaning that animals need to grow fast, and carcass yields must be high so that in the end Old McDonald can deliver you the "best" product at the lowest cost (neither the animals' health nor yours really matters here). And how do they make efficiency happen? By administering hormones.

A hormone is an incredibly important and volatile regulatory substance produced in an organism naturally and transported in body fluids such as blood to trigger specific cells into action. There are many types of hormones, all with specific functions, but for the moment, you need only be concerned with the reproductive and maturation stimulants.

Growth hormones were first approved for use on beef cattle in 1954. Currently, six hormones are approved for use on cattle (use in poultry was banned in the 1950s and now federal regulations prohibit their use in pigs as well). The hormones administered to cattle are typically packaged in a pellet that is surgically implanted behind the ear when they check into the feedlot "hotel." These include estrogen, progesterone, testosterone, zeranol, trenbolone, and melengestrol. When administered to cattle, the naturally occurring hormone levels can increase seven to twenty times. That means that your meat is pumped up. And let's not forget the artificially made (and genetically modified) recombinant bovine growth hormone (rBGH) that increases milk yield in lactating cows, compliments of Monsanto.

According to the FDA:

These drugs increase the animals' growth rate, the efficiency by which they convert the feed they eat into meat, and the leanness of their meat. The FDA approved these drugs only after extensive studies have shown that the food from the treated animals is safe for people to eat, and that the drugs do not harm the treated animal or the environment. The drugs also have to work as intended.[2]

Using scientific data, the FDA establishes acceptable safe limits for hormones in meat. A safe level for human consumption is one that would be expected to have no effect in humans based on extensive scientific study and review.

I don't know about you, but I have a difficult time dealing with my own hormone issues. I have no interest in taking on additional hormone hardships from another source, even if they are deemed all right by regulators.

On Ractopamine

But wait, that's not all. There is another drug, beta-agonist ractopamine, being widely used among livestock, most notably cattle and pork, that remains "under the radar" and has a stunning list of side effects related to the cardiovascular and musculoskeletal systems.

According to Andrew Gunther of AWA, records from the FDA's Center for Veterinary Medicine reveal that within a few years of ractopamine's approval for commercial use, the manufacturer (Eli Lilly) had received hundreds of reports from farmers and veterinarians about sickened pigs. Gunther also notes that more recent data released by the FDA reveals that since ractopamine was approved for pigs in 1999, over 160,000 have suffered from adverse effects including hyperactivity, trembling, broken limbs, inability to walk, and death. Yet ractopamine remains in use in the United States while the European Union, China, and more than one hundred other countries have banned its use.[3]

And get this: A study posted on the National Institutes of Health's Toxicology Data Network looked at the dose-dependent effects of ractopamine on humans. The study showed that as the dose slowly increased, so did heart rate and cardiac output[4]—meaning that your heart had to work a little harder to keep you ticking. Exercise, not unnecessary additives in your food, should do that. Although this is only *one* study on a small group of individuals, it's enough for me to say no to this drug.

Why They Are "Bad"

Thanks to organizations like GRACE and the folks at Animal Welfare Approved, info on animals can be at anyone's fingertips. Some researchers believe that hormonal residues, measurable levels of which are present at slaughter in the muscle, fat, liver, kidneys, and other organ meats of livestock, contribute to premature puberty in young girls—an occurrence associated with higher risk for breast cancer later in life. Remnants are also thought to cause lower sperm count in boys. So it seems that these stimulants can disrupt hormone balance, natural development, and reproduction as well as possibly causing cancers.

rBGH, best beware. The FDA will tell you it is safe (like all other hormones), but the real concern lies in the fact that this hormone may trigger the production of another hormone (remember, these substances are the *real regulators* in any organism), insulin-like growth factor (IGF), which can in turn mimic the effects of human growth hormone. And in cows treated with rBGH, there is ten times more IGF than in other milk. In 2004, the *Journal of Clinical Oncology*, the *European Journal of Clinical Nutrition*, and *PLOS Biology* all published studies linking high levels of IGF with increased velocity of natural development and multiple cancers.[5]

Growth-promoting hormones not only remain in the meat and dairy you consume but also get excreted in manure. According to GRACE:

Scientists are increasingly concerned about the environmental impacts of [growth-promoting] hormone residues as [they leak] from manure into the environment, contaminating soil and surface groundwater. Aquatic ecosystems are particularly vulnerable to hormone residues and recent studies have demonstrated that exposure to hormones has a substantial effect on the gender and reproductive capacity of fish.[6]

Irrespective of the fact that the European Union rejects hormone use in cattle, ended imports of hormone-treated beef in 1988, and wants nothing tainted from the United States, this country continues to turn a blind eye to the damage being done to animals, human health, and the environment.

While the FDA *expects* that the hormones have no effect on your health and the environment based on "extensive" scientific evidence, questions and controversies have existed for decades and aren't effectively being answered and remedied.

The Better for You Alternatives

Since hormones are not used in poultry and pork, no worries there. But when it comes to cattle, pick and choose wisely. Use the same guidelines suggested for antibiotics.

Love the local farmer (and I surely buy from her or him), but I prefer the ones with third-party verification like AWA or Certified Humane. USDA Organic is also a good option. Don't necessarily buy into that label lingo like "cage free" because sadly, these labels are confusing at best. Chapter 11 will help get the record straight. And don't forget Meatless Mondays.

When buying dairy products, whether milk, yogurt, or cheese, *always* go organic if you can. Otherwise, go with brands like Applegate Farms (for cheese) that assure you that no rBGH was used and are hopefully keeping their promise. If you have questions about the product you are about to purchase, pick up your cell phone while in the dairy aisle and call to find some answers. You have a right to know.

A Fishy Situation

The summer of 2013 was a good one. Tipped off by a friend about Dock to Dish, a new community-supported fishery (that is, a shoreside community of people collaborating with the local fishermen to have access to the truly fresh, local catch of the day), I immediately reached out to cofounder Sean Barrett. And not only did I gain weekly access to incredibly delicious, local, sustainable seafood, but I also learned so much more about the not-so-simple side of everything fish.

For starters, as reported by FishWatch (part of the National Oceanic and Atmospheric Administration [NOAA]), "The U.S. imports over 91% of its seafood, about half of which is from aquaculture."[7] Equally astonishing is that a significant portion of our imported wild seafood was actually caught here, but then shipped overseas for processing—fileting, deboning, and packaging—because it is cheaper. Some of it is then *reimported* for sale as "local" seafood (even though it has traveled as far as China and India and back). And according to Marianne Cufone, environmental attorney and executive director of Recirculating Farms Coalition, an NGO that supports the development of eco-efficient farms that use clean, recycled water as the basis to grow food, "less than 2% of your imported seafood is inspected for 'filth'" (as in mouse, rat, and human hair and insects).[8] Food traveling great distances is handled by many, thus cleanliness can be an issue.

In addition, when fish is sent overseas for processing, not only is it often frozen but also chemicals such as sulfur dioxide and sodium tripolyphosphate (STPP), a chemical with GRAS status that can make your sea creatures appear firmer and glossier (and exposure can be dangerous if inhaled, as noted by the FDA), may be added to your seafood to keep it looking fresh (scallops and shrimp are commonly soaked in STPP). Cufone adds, "labeling requirements are complicated, confusing and not well enforced. Some of these chemicals might appear on a label—or they might not [other than sulfur dioxide and some other sulfites at levels above 10 parts per million]. For example, there is no requirement to let consumers know STPP was used, and this can make seafood look fresher than it is."[9] Best that you presume that your fish has been frozen, thawed, and refrozen (and has added preservatives) *unless* it says "never been frozen" or something similar; and inquire about chemicals. Cufone suggests, "If your fish is caught and processed in the U.S. (the USDA requires Country of Labeling Origin on seafood, with some exceptions) then it's more likely that your fish has only been frozen and thawed once, so it's your better choice."[10] As I always tell my clients, unless you live in a coastal community and know your fishermen, your best bet is frozen fish caught and processed in the United States.

According to FishWatch, aquaculture, "also known as fish or shellfish farming, refers to the breeding, rearing and harvesting of plants and animals in all types of water environments including ponds, rivers, lakes and the ocean."[11] Essentially, your fishy friends are raised in controlled environments (rather than the wild), just as cattle and poultry are raised. If done right, aquaculture alleviates the ever-increasing demands on ocean waters; while the farms provide, the ocean wild can replenish. There are two types of aquaculture—open systems and closed systems (either recirculating or nonrecirculating).

While some fish and shellfish are farmed with health in mind (mainly, the recirculating sort), most live just as your livestock do—in overcrowded quarters, often alongside dead and decaying fish and fish waste. As a result, sickness abounds, and the swimmers are often treated with antibiotics so they can better withstand the stress. As per Food and Water Watch: "Residues of these antibiotics travel with seafood from their tank to your table. Chloramphenicol, penicillin and other drugs used in production can pose serious health risks to consumers who may become susceptible to antibiotic-resistant bacteria. For the many people with allergies to antibiotics, contaminated seafood can cause unexpected allergic reactions. The Food and Drug Administration (FDA) stated that clear scientific evidence indicates that the use of these drugs and chemicals in raising seafood can lead to an increased antimicrobial resistance in human pathogens (stronger germs that are resistant to our medicines) and that prolonged exposure to some of these chemicals has been shown to cause cancer."[12]

In the case of hormones, there is unavoidable runoff in the natural habitat from stimulants given to livestock—so whether fish are wild or from a farm, contaminants can be ever present. Plus, according to Food and Water Watch, hormones are being administered to fish in many hatcheries (where farm-raised fish begin their lives) because life in captivity means fish don't successfully breed and thus need a little help. The hormones of choice are chorionic gonadotropin, a human hormone and common fertility drug, and luteinizing hormone-releasing hormone. Chorionic gonadotropin "can increase the risk of multiple pregnancy, premature puberty, and ovarian enlargement and cysts." The FDA does not regularly test fish for residues of the hormone, nor does it take any other regulatory action to enforce limits. Currently, there are no national aquaculture standards in the United States, but individual states do have some mandates, though typically with little oversight and monitoring. So sadly, farmed fish can be quite a scuffle.

How to navigate fish and shellfish? If you can't get it from your fishermen, whether through a Dock to Dish–like model or your local fishmonger who sources directly from the fishing boats:

1. Find out where it comes from—as in the United States (good) or overseas (not as good).
2. Is it wild (good, if from uncontaminated waters and responsibly fished) or farmed (closed, recirculating is your best bet)? For some shellfish—like clams, mussels, or oysters—farming in open water can be okay. Shellfish are filter feeders, meaning they suck in water, eat tiny particles, then release the water. So they can actually help clean the waters in which they are raised. Look for hand collected, raked, or rope or bag grown.
3. To avoid the chemicals, since labeling is a bit of a nightmare, it's best to ask questions to *hopefully ensure* that chemicals were not added. Find the fishmonger who can address your inquiries.

To learn more about the specific ins and outs of your fish, Monterey Bay Aquarium created Seafood Watch, a consumers' guide and smartphone app for choosing seafood that is healthier for the oceans and you (more on this in chapter 14). Also, NOAA keeps tabs on everything fish-related, especially the wild sort, so if you want further insight, it's the place to go.

CHAPTER 10

Genetically Modified Organisms (GMOs)*

While having dinner at a reputable restaurant near my home, I noticed a dish offering "Corn-Fed Skirt Steak." Why this restaurant chose to honor corn is baffling, as it is surely *not* something to boast about. Knowing what you *now* know about cattle, how they are raised, and what they really should be eating, would you want to eat corn-fed beef? I get that for many there is no other option so you have to pick and choose your battles, but let me add a little insult to injury here. I can pretty much promise you that the corn this moo was eating in his accelerated life was genetically modified, as roughly 88 percent of the U.S. corn crop is altered by science.

As you now understand, I have spent the better part of my life analyzing, or overanalyzing, everything food. You have read about a host of my concerns regarding the food system, but to me, there is nothing more infuriating than genetic modification.

Folks, you have been a science experiment for the biotech industry without even knowing it. GMOs have never been tested for *true* safety for human consumption; rather they have been presumed safe by their creators and your government for decades.

*Although health, safety and environmental regulations are in place, they are very weak and loosely regulated by the U.S. government.

What They Are

Genetically modified organisms (GMOs) are plants or animals created through gene-splicing techniques (also called biotechnology). This technology merges DNA from different species, creating potentially unstable combinations of plant, animal, bacterial, and viral genes that cannot occur in nature (or in traditional crossbreeding). While almost all commercial GMOs are engineered mainly to tolerate direct application of herbicide and/or to produce an insecticide, Monsanto (one of the leading biotech companies) claims that the world needs genetically modified food for three reasons:

1. to produce more food because the world's population is growing
2. to produce better food that's more nutritious
3. to find ways to make the process of growing food more efficient and aligned with environmental needs, so farmers use less water and land and better use things like fertilizer, herbicides, and pesticides.[1]

Ultimately this is what the world of biotech wants you to believe. But in reality, there is plenty of food to go around. According to the United Nations' Food and Agriculture Organization (FAO), a recent study revealed that:

[R]oughly one third of all food production worldwide gets lost or wasted in the food production and consumption systems. Almost half of this quantity is the result of retailers and consumers in industrialized regions discarding food that is fit for consumption. The total quantity wasted is about 300 million tons, which is more than the total net food production of Sub-Saharan Africa. It would be sufficient to feed the estimated 900 million people hungry in the world.[2]

So is genetically modified food necessary, or do people just need to be more conscientious about how they produce, distribute, and consume the world's food supply?

Now let's move on to Monsanto's second argument in support of GMOs: to produce better, more nutritious food. Golden rice was engineered as a source of beta-carotene, a precursor to vitamin A, in order to address the dietary deficiencies of many children and pregnant women in regions where rice is a staple food. Altering the genes of the rice was seen as a simple and less expensive alternative to supplying the undernourished with vitamin supplements or more green vegetables and animal products. Supporters of this endeavor suggest that engineering golden rice is like fluoridating water (as is common in the United States) or adding iodine to salt. I, however, contend that a comparison does not exist here—altering the genetic makeup of a food is far different from adding something to a food.

This golden child has not yet been approved for sale, as many questions still remain about its true safety (and whether it can even solve the deficiency problem). In 2009, while research was being conducted at an American university to test the safety and set protocols for human trials of this rice, a group of twenty-two international scientists and experts expressed great concern. As noted by the Institute for Science and Society, a center of excellence in science and technology at Nottingham University:

> There is now a large body of evidence that shows that GM crop/food production is highly prone to inadvertent and unpredictable pleiotropic [producing multiple] effects, which can result in health damaging effects when GM food products are fed to animals. More specifically, our greatest concern is that this rice, which is engineered to overproduce beta carotene, has never been tested in animals, and there is extensive medical literature showing that retinoids that can be derived from beta carotene are both toxic and cause birth defects.[3]

Despite concern from Nottingham, in 2012 this American university published an article in the *American Journal of Clinical Nutrition* stating that "[r]ecruitment processes and protocol were approved" for the testing of rice on humans.[4] One human trial to note occurred through this American university and resulted in the lead scientist being punished for violating university and U.S. federal rules on human research. As of 2014, this golden grain has neither been tested for safety nor adequately tested for its ability to make vitamin A. Thus it is still not ready for commercial release globally.[5] I suspect that the amount of time and money that has gone into golden rice since it was first developed in the 1990s hasn't made it "a simple and less expensive alternative."

Lastly, the claim of "improving agriculture" by better use of things like fertilizer, herbicides, and pesticides is absurd. Monsanto is not only the leading producer of genetically modified seeds but also the prime producer and pusher of the herbicide glyphosate (the active ingredient in the Roundup brand) that is used worldwide. Is this company really looking to improve agriculture or their bottom line?

The commercial sale of GMOs began in 1994 with the introduction of the Flavr Savr tomato by Calgene. This tomato was genetically modified to slow the ripening process—preventing the tomato from rotting too soon. The FDA stated that special labeling for these modified tomatoes was *not* necessary because they had the essential characteristics of nonmodified tomatoes, there was no evidence of health risks, and the nutritional content was unchanged. While the Flavr Savr tomato no longer exists, many other crops are genetically modified or have a high risk of being genetically modified according to the most recent data from the Non-GMO Project,[6] and the USDA.[7] They include the following:

1. Alfalfa (as much as 90 percent)
2. Canola (roughly 90 percent of the U.S. crop)
3. Corn (roughly 93 percent of the U.S. crop)
4. Cotton—from which cottonseed oil is derived (roughly 96 percent of the U.S. crop)
5. Papaya (most of the Hawaiian crop)
6. Soy (roughly 94 percent of the U.S. crop)

7. Sugar beets (roughly 99 percent of the U.S. crop)[8]
8. Zucchini and yellow squash (25,000 acres' worth)

And it doesn't stop there. Be wary of animals for food production as, more often than not, what they eat is composed of GMO ingredients (like corn). And remember, you are not only what you eat, *but also what they ate.* Several plants, including chard, beets (like the common red and yellow), rutabaga, turnip, acorn squash, flax, and rice, are regularly monitored because cross-contamination with GMO crops has been known to occur. But what I also want you to grasp is that a large portion of the ingredients in food products—ranging from breads and cereals to snacks, sweets, and beverages—are most likely derived from those GMO sources. The following are a *few* of these ingredients:

1. Amino acids—found in supplements and protein powders
2. Ascorbic acid—also called vitamin C and used as a preservative in many foods
3. Aspartame—found in NutraSweet and Equal, as well as many "sugar-free" products
4. Beet sugar—found as a sweetener in many beverages
5. Canola oil—found in many snacks such as chips, crackers, nut mixes, and sweets
6. Cottonseed oil—found in many snacks such as chips, crackers, nut mixes, and sweets
7. Flavorings (both natural and artificial)
8. High-fructose corn syrup (corn syrup)—found in most packaged foods such as cereals, snacks, and sweets
9. Hydrolyzed vegetable protein and textured vegetable protein—both found in many vegetarian packaged foods such as soups, chili, and fake meats
10. Maltodextrins—a common starchy food additive found in many packaged foods including snacks and sweets
11. Molasses—if it comes from sugar beets

12. Monosodium glutamate (MSG)—that flavor enhancer found in many packaged soups and flavored grain products and commonly used in Chinese fast food
13. Soy protein isolate—found in many "high-protein" products like shakes, bars, and cereals, and in many snacks like chips and even cookies
14. Soy sauce
15. Sugar—if it comes from sugar beets
16. Vitamins—whether in supplement form or in your food
17. Xanthan gum—found in many packaged foods from soups to snacks

So now you know that a large percentage of the food you eat is somehow touched by genetic modification. And another thing, GMO fish are in the pipeline (see sidebar, "GMO and Animals," page 93). Sadly, GMOs are not going away anytime soon.

Why They Are "Bad"

Let me start with this—while there is really *no evidence* whatsoever supporting the safety of GMOs for human consumption, as no long-term animal studies have been conducted (although partial research does exist from the corporations that create and profit from them), there is *some* evidence suggesting that dangers clearly prevail.

On January 17, 2013, internationally recognized plant pathologist (and former professor at Purdue University) Dr. Don Huber expressed concerns about Roundup Ready corn and soy (both GMO crops).[9] A little background: Roundup Ready crops are bioengineered to resist the herbicide Roundup, meaning that when Roundup is sprayed to kill ever-present weeds, the GMO crops are sure to withstand the herbicide. Both the seeds for these crops and the herbicide, whose active ingredient is glyphosate, are compliments of Monsanto. While glyphosate has its toxicity issues, levels in use are deemed safe by the EPA.

Dr. Huber wrote a letter to Tom Vilsack, U.S. secretary of agriculture, warning of a new pathogen in this Roundup Ready corn and soy and its possible link to plant and animal diseases—like sudden death syndrome in soy and Goss's wilt (a bacteria) in corn, as well as infertility and spontaneous abortions in cows—that are reaching epidemic proportions. He urged the USDA to participate in a multiagency investigation and moratorium on plantings of such crops until their possible threat to the health of plants and animals, *including humans*, can be ruled out. Despite Huber's plea, the Obama administration approved two new Roundup Ready crops for planting less than three weeks later.

But there is more—because of the widespread use of Roundup, a "super weed" that is resistant to glyphosate has been born. As a result, farmers have no choice but to turn to increasingly toxic chemicals. And as it turns out, one of these chemicals being used more extensively on crops like corn, 2,4-dichlorophenoxyacetic acid, was a major ingredient in Agent Orange— a chemical that was used in the Vietnam War and caused the death or maiming of more than four hundred thousand people and birth defects in an estimated half million infants.

And get this—genetically modified seeds are patentable. Thus, biotech companies are allowed to restrict their use. These GMO seeds inevitably find their way into neighboring farms that are not using GMO seeds, mainly due to contamination of seed supply. As a result, biotech companies are given the power to sue these innocent farmers—threatening them, their businesses, and their livelihood.

Can it get much worse? Well, sadly there is no law that requires labeling of GMOs. In November 2012, California attempted to pass Proposition 37—a law that would have required all food with GMOs to be labeled as such in the state. This proposition was met with great resistance not only by Monsanto but also Big Ag and Big Food (industry giants like Coca-Cola, ConAgra, General Mills, Kraft, Kellogg's, Pepsi, and Unilever, which produce both conventional brands and even some of the healthier ones on the market today). While nearly 47 percent of all Californians voted in favor of Prop 37, the big guys won. With roughly $46 million invested in radio and TV campaigns alone (to coerce and celebrate GMOs), how could they not? In the end, your health came second to industry's bottom line. But the good news is that this single state's movement sparked a nationwide Right to Know GMO campaign. Individual states are working toward GMO labeling laws, and some, like Vermont*, Maine, and Connecticut, are succeeding; hopefully others are not far behind.

The Better for You Alternatives

Whether you choose to eat anything altered by science is up to you. I truly honor what people can and will do. But I would be foolish not to give you the tools to navigate GMOs and exercise your right to know.

Even if your food is 100 percent organic, it can still be contaminated with GMOs. Right now testing for genetically modified ingredients in your food has limitations, so impostors can't be adequately identified to ensure that your food is GMO-free. Though I will leave you with this: *Hopefully* your organic food does not contain GMOs.

As not everyone can travel the "organic highway," the Non-GMO Project launched a certification program, so that when you see their logo, you can feel safe (despite noted testing limitations) that your eats are not altered. In fact, the Non-GMO Project has a great Shopping Guide that you can download to your smartphone as a convenient resource (more on this in chapter 15). Sometimes, even if a product does not have the blue, green, and orange stamp of approval, it may still be labeled GMO-free (I recommend inquiring further, as Non-GMO Project is fast becoming the standard).

*In June 2014, the Grocery Manufacturers Association (GMA), the voice of more than 300 *leading* food manufacturers in the United States (in other words, Big Food), the Snack Food Association, the International Dairy Foods Association, and the National Association of Manufacturers sued the state of Vermont claiming that their new mandatory GMO labeling law violates free speech. Very simply, Vermont fought for their right to know, won, and the big guys are not happy. The state expected this pushback and is prepared to zealously continue the fight. To be continued....

And if you can't manage either, try to avoid the plants and the ingredients that are bioengineered, as noted earlier in this chapter. This is a tough task for sure, but one that can at least minimize your exposure.

As far as exercising your right to know goes, check out Just Label It, an NGO that will keep you updated and informed on everything GMO. And you can take action locally or globally through one of these incredible food justice dynamos:

- Center for Food Safety
- Consumers Union
- Food and Water Watch
- Food Democracy Now
- Institute for Responsible Technology
- Organic Consumers Association
- The Non-GMO Project

A student of mine recently asked, "Knowing all that you know about food, how do you actually eat and enjoy?"

My answer: "With all that I know, I have learned how to navigate this food system gone awry, but I still have to be realistic and understand that I can't be pure all of the time. We can all only do the best we can with what we have."

So, get educated, make better choices, and vote with your fork!

GMO and Animals

AquaBounty Technologies is developing advanced hybrid salmon, trout, and tilapia designed to grow faster than their conventional counterparts. And guess what: AquaAdvantage Salmon will be the very first *genetically modified animal intended for human consumption* to hit your supermarket shelves, thanks to the FDA, whose "preliminary finding is that an approval of this application, under the specific conditions proposed in the application, would not have a significant impact on the U.S. environment."[10] Basically the genetic engineering of the eggs would take place in Canada, and then they would be shipped to Panama, where they would be raised in inland tanks. Once killed and processed in Panama, the "fish" will be shipped to the United States, all ready for you to enjoy. Unfortunately there is really no way for you to know if the salmon you will be buying in a store or eating in a restaurant is one that has been altered because there are no mandatory labeling laws. But the good news is that as of March 2014, nine thousand stores across the nation, including Kroger and Safeway, have rejected this new "fish" for sale. But it could be in your store in the near future, so shop salmon with caution.

The Altered Apple

The Arctic Apple is another one of biotech's new brainchildren. Finally the perfect Pink Lady, Red Delicious, or Granny Smith. But is this truly the apple a day that can keep the doctor away? Hmmm . . .

The apple won't turn brown when you cut into it. In fact, it will look fresh and edible all the time. It will be perfect on the outside, and white, white, white on the inside. And soon, fast-food restaurants, as well as school *cafeterias* that feed your little loved ones, could be serving up this altered apple.

So, what's the big deal? While food isn't perfect (we live in an imperfect world), the biotech industry wants to make food infallible. By doing so, the food supply is more predictable—crops won't get eaten by pests, will tolerate droughts, and won't freeze if it gets too chilly—and predictability means profit. So biotech plays with nature by altering genes to create "indestructible" eats.

Based on the Arctic Apple's website, courtesy of Okanagan Specialty Fruits, this is the deal:[11]

All apples undergo enzymatic browning due to a chemical reaction after cell injury, whether by bruising, biting, or cutting the apple. Arctic apples don't undergo this enzymatic browning because the genes (or switches, as I like to say) responsible for the browning are turned off (or silenced) by a bunch of scientists in a lab. While gene silencing is a natural process that all plants (and animals) use to control expression of their genes in *nature*, the Arctic Apple's genes are manipulated in a lab. Sounds pretty Frankenstein to me.

The genetically engineered seeds (where the genetic material lives) are grown into plantlets that grow in a tree nursery until they are ready to be transplanted to an orchard, just like other commercial apple tree seedlings. Once in the orchard, they behave just as other apple trees do—they grow, flower and bear fruit, and react to pests and weather in the same way. As for pesticides, the Arctic Apple is no different from any apple (unless certified organic)—they are both bathed in pesticides. And as a result, they will consistently top the Environmental Working Group's Dirty Dozen™ for the staggering array of chemicals found on them (just as their unengineered, nonorganic counterparts do now).

But, according to biotech, they are not taking genes from another species and inserting them into the genetic material of the apple (like most other GMOs). Rather they are altering what is already in the apple. So what's the harm?

1. This new science experiment is basically an untested genetic technology—isn't it enough that you have been lab rats for biotech for decades without knowing it?
2. Despite biotech's claim that genetically engineered "matter" is destroyed by human digestion (and thus not harmful to you), these manipulated genes do find their way into your digestive systems and bloodstream (you are what you eat) and could potentially damage vital human genes.

I don't know about you, but given this info, I sure as heck wouldn't want to take a chance with my health or that of my kids. I would rather eat an apple than an apple anomaly. Your best bet is to go organic for all apples.

There's More: Wheat and Mutagenesis

For years I was sure that GMO wheat was rampant in the food supply. Good news, it technically is not genetically modified. But for decades now it has undergone a process called mutagenesis. Suspicious? Well, you should be. Mutagenesis, a process of exposing seeds to chemicals or radiation in order to generate mutants with desirable traits (prior to breeding with other plants), has been used on wheat for decades. It is not unlike genetic engineering in that it may produce unknown allergens and toxins in food. Sadly, all the work to label GMOs won't touch mutagenesis. In fact, mutagenic wheat is allowed in organic food. Bottom line, your food can be seriously tainted, so aim to understand the issues (even if just a little bit) so you can better navigate your eats.

As far as how to navigate wheat, I think I may be without words here because for one, most commercial wheat undergoes mutagenesis, and second, it is currently permissible in organics. But the good thing is that you can take action on this issue and many others by connecting with one of the Food Policy, Safety and Accountability organizations in Appendix E, "Redeemable Resources."

The Last Word on the Top-Rated Terminators

If you are buying a car, do you thoroughly research the brand, whether Toyota or Chevy? The answer is probably yes. You scour the Internet, prepare a list of questions to take to multiple car dealers, and test-drive to utter insanity. Hey, if you're going to spend that amount of money, you better know what you are getting yourself into.

The funny thing is that in the three decades that I have been into food, I have rarely met a person who gives the same amount of thought to what they put in their body as they do to the car that they aim to buy. Is a car really more important than your health? The answer is no. But the question remains: Why don't most people act otherwise?

The super-simple answer is that food marketing has faked you out. You want to believe everything food producers tell you, whether through ads, packaging, or even those in-store product pushes. It's a heck of a lot easier to grab and go. And so long as a food is low in fat, sugar, and calories, you're sold. Well think again, because sadly, labels lie. And your health is not only about the grams of fat and sugar, or calories—it's also about the ingredients and where they came from. On top of that, you trust a government that does a below-average job of regulating food. Well, learn how to be your own advocate and take action with *What the Fork*—I am here to help you do something more than just read about it!

Pantry Rehab

I don't wear a white coat or carry a prescription pad. I don't have an office where those seeking a food solution to prevent or manage illness come to see me. Instead, we meet in the comfort of their homes to chat (and eventually chew). Step one is an extensive evaluation in which one of my first questions is, "What are your goals in working with me?" Nine out of ten times, weight loss is numero uno on the list (whether that person needs to lose weight or not).

We gab about personal health history, family health history, relationship to food (as in what their diet was like growing up, who cooked, etc.); we touch on exercise and dive into what's eaten in a day before I once again ask, "Can you rethink what your goals are in working with me?"

And most of the time the answer is something like, "To gain a better understanding of what a healthy diet is for me [and my family] and to shift my eating habits to support my overall health." Hallelujah! And then there is a pause before they ask, "Do you think that I will still lose weight?"

After years of working with people from all walks of life, I can tell you this: With the *right* help and a *real commitment* on your part, you can get healthy and stay healthy. *What the Fork* is neither a crash diet nor a cleanse; rather, it is a guide to spotlight what you are eating and to give you tools to transition everything edible (or even just one or two things) from the ground up. Because when you're finished with those fads, you go right back to the same old unhealthy structure you came from. And the cycle repeats.

But I am here to change that. While I am in my clients' homes, descending on their kitchens and peeking through their pantry, fridge, and freezer is unavoidable. Funny enough, over the years, I've found that a person would rather I look in their bedroom or bathroom than at their food. As you probably can guess, food choice speaks volumes and contributes valuable insight into each client, ultimately giving me the tools to help them restructure their eats. Hey, if I don't know what's broken, I can't help fix it.

Consider *What the Fork* to be your personal guide to a do-it-yourself (DIY) pantry rehab (fridge and freezer included). But before we go there, I need to give you the lowdown on food labels. After all, they are a language unto themselves, and you need to know how to read and understand them before you make those game-changing rehab decisions.

CHAPTER 11

Food Labels 101

Bottom line: Consider yourself bound to get brainwashed if you don't know how to vet food labels, whether Nutrition Facts, ingredient lists, health claims, and the funny (and not so funny) label lingo. Being skeptical about sustenance, even if ever so slightly, goes a long way.

A diabetic client of mine loves chocolate. Instead of moderating his chocolate intake, he would opt for a small bar daily whose label boasted "safe for diabetics" and "sugar-free" (the sugar substitute of choice being sorbitol, a sugar alcohol noted in sidebar "On Other Sugar Substitutes," page 40). A few weeks into his habit, he developed bloating and pooping problems. Sugar alcohols, if consumed in excess (and even in moderation for some), can not only cause gastrointestinal upset but also act as a laxative. The moral of the story: The flashy banners on a product, even the Nutrition Facts, don't tell the whole story of your food; the ingredient lists do. As for my client, he now eats one to two squares of dark chocolate (with very little added sugar) per day, and feels fine and pretty darn happy.

If you are like him, you have most likely fallen prey to the meticulous marketing behind food. Don't get me wrong, I do care about the calories, fat, sodium, and sugar content of food (especially when working with people with illness), but the way I see it, it's the actual ingredients in a product that impact your health—what they are and where they come from.

Before you begin your DIY Pantry Rehab, I want to give you the CliffsNotes version of what all those facts, lists, claims, and lingo on your labels *really* mean, so you know how to navigate your nourishment. You would hope that the labels tell all, but they truly don't. In fact, they often mislead, so let's get you educated.

The Nutrition Facts Label as You Know It

Most people think that the Nutrition Facts is *the* scoop on your food. Think again. While it is required on most packaged products, it's only part of the story.

The foundation for the Facts is the "Percent Daily Value" listed on the right side of the label. It is essentially a guide to the nutrients in *one* serving of food. According to the FDA, the agency behind the Daily Values (DVs), the DVs are based on a 2,000-calorie diet for *healthy* adults. Keep in mind that plenty of people consume less than 2,000 calories in a day, and even

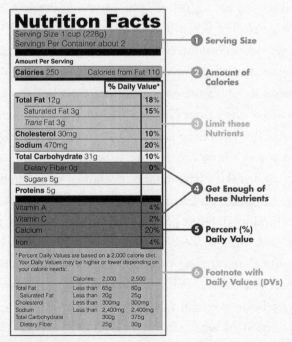

For educational purposes only. This label does not meet the labeling requirements described in 21 CFR 101.9.

more consume far beyond. And a large percentage of the population is not so healthy. So the DVs are just an average.

On the actual label, this is basically what you see: the serving size (is it 8 ounces or 16 ounces?); the calories in *one* serving of the product; and the "skinny" on fat (unsaturated = good fat, saturated = "bad" fat, and trans = really bad fat), cholesterol, sodium, carbohydrate (including fiber and sugar), and protein. Last but not least are the Daily Values of vitamins and minerals in your food, although they typically are not much to shout about for anything too processed.

Now this is where it gets super confusing: I once picked up a reputable tea beverage that had a serving size of 8 fluid ounces. Sugar was 12 grams. I was pretty psyched—a seemingly low-sugar tea drink. But, think again— there were *two servings per container*, meaning that I forgot to multiply the Daily Values by two. And who drinks only half a bottle of a ready-to-drink beverage? Buyer, beware.

But there is some good news—the Nutrition Facts makeover has begun. As printed in the *Federal Register*, the daily journal of the U.S. government, on March 3, 2014: "The Food and Drug Administration (FDA, the Agency, or we) is proposing to amend its labeling regulations for conventional foods and dietary supplements to provide updated nutrition information on the label to assist consumers in maintaining healthy dietary practices."[1]

The New and "Improved" Nutrition Facts Label

So what does this mean for you in the end? Lisa Young, PhD, RDN, CDN, notable nutritionist, portion-size expert, and author of *The Portion Teller Plan*, suggests that one of the most important changes is serving size, making it larger and more realistic: ". . . a pint of ice cream that currently has four servings per pint (each serving is ½ cup), will have two servings for the new proposed label (each serving size will increase to 1 cup). The calories listed will, therefore, also increase. If a ½ cup serving of ice cream contains 200 calories, with the new 1 cup serving size, the label will now display 400 calories."[2]

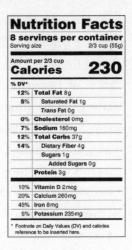

According to Young, "The serving sizes will be more realistic and reflect what people really eat. Many people today just glance at the calories and think that whatever amount they eat is a serving. For the ice cream example, a consumer reading food labels will now see 400 calories displayed instead of 200 calories. This may mean that you would think twice before scarfing down the entire pint."[3]

This *potential* consumption clarity won't change overnight, but rather will roll out over the course of the next couple of years.

What the Fork to Do

1. Focus on "serving size" and "servings per container," always understanding that the numbers and percentages are typically based on *one* serving *only*.

2. Keep an eye out for fat content, knowing that it's "best" if your bite has 5 percent or less per serving. Fat content of 20 percent is considered way high.

3. Go for zero trans fats at all times. Remember, these man-made fats are the real culprits, more so than saturated fat and sugar. And do note that even if the Facts say no trans fats, they can still be present in your food, just at a quantity of less than 0.5 grams. So always refer to your ingredient lists to get the better truth.

4. Watch out for sodium, again knowing that it's best to stay in that 5 percent ballpark. The Dietary Guidelines for Americans (science-based recommendations from the U.S. Department of Health and Human Services' Office of Disease Prevention and

Health Promotion) state that sodium intake should not exceed 2,300 milligrams (mg) per day for Americans age two and over. According to the Mayo Clinic, the average person is sucking down around 3,400 mg of sodium daily. Sodium (and lots of it) lives in processed foods. And if you are adding it to your eats, a single teaspoon of table salt contains 2,325 mg of saltiness.

5. As far as sugar is concerned, my general rule of thumb is to keep it as low as possible. The American Heart Association suggests that men limit *added* sugar to 36 grams (9 teaspoons) per day, and women to 24 grams (6 teaspoons) per day. I am not talking about sugar in fruit or other carbohydrates, but rather the sugar that is oh-so-generously added to almost everything processed. To translate, one bottle of a very popular sports drink has roughly 32.5 grams of sugar.

As for all the other info on the Facts, I don't mean to brush them aside, but they don't hold a heck of a lot of weight for me. I think the Nutrition Facts are confusing at best and do a half-assed job of talking about the real nutrition in food. It's the ingredients that offer the necessary narrative.

Ingredient Lists

Do you focus on the Facts, noting calories and fat, salt, and sugar content, then decide if you are going in for the product purchase? Or do you give them a quick glance, then swiftly slide through the ingredient list? Either way, the deal maker or breaker is most likely the Facts. Why? Most people are conditioned to think that calories, fat, salt, and sugar are the ultimate determinants of health. Sorry to burst your bubble, but that is just not true.

You can have a low-calorie and low-sugar product that relies on chemical sweeteners for taste appeal like many of those diet beverages on the market. And believe it or not, you can have a low-fat product loaded with sugar (often the sugar replaces the fat because technically sugar has no fat).

Salad dressings are a prime example of a low-fat condiment with excess sugar. These are just some of the Big Food tricks that, time and again, sucker you. But as we've learned so far, low-fat and sugar-free aren't the be-all and end-all of healthy.

So, this is the deal: The ingredient list (as you will see in the following example) truly tells the story of your food. So skim the Facts and investigate the ingredients. I don't balk at products with fat, salt, and sugar (all inherent in packaged foods). And yes, I eat packaged foods just like you. But I do some heavy-duty scrutinizing to determine the real story of anything edible. Let me break it down for you.

MAINSTREAM CRACKER INGREDIENT LIST Enriched Bleached Wheat Flour (Bleached Flour, Malted Barley Flour, Niacin, Iron, Thiamin, Mononitrate, Riboflavin, Folic Acid), Vegetable Oil (contains one or more of the following oils: Cottonseed Oil, Palm Oil, Soybean Oil), Dextrose, Water, Sugar, High Fructose Corn Syrup, Modified Food Starch (Corn and/or Wheat), Contains 2% or less of the following: Eggs, Nonfat Milk, Glycerin, Soy Flour, Corn Syrup Solids, Leavening (Sodium Acid Pyrophosphate, Baking Soda, Sodium Aluminum Phosphate), Preservatives (Potassium Sorbate, Sodium Propionate, Calcium Propionate), Salt, Natural and Artificial Flavor, Mono- and Diglycerides, Soy Lecithin, Spices, Tapioca Starch, Wheat Starch, Artificial Color, Cellulose Gum, Guar Gum, Karaya Gum, colored with extracts of Annatto and Turmeric.

1. **Enriched bleached wheat flour:** Because most of the vitamins inherent in the wheat are stripped away during processing, food makers enrich the flour with these vital micronutrients. Then, like that isn't enough, they add a chemical bleaching agent (such as chlorine—though it is not permitted in Europe) to make the flour appear whiter and more "suitable" for baking. I try to avoid "enriched bleached" anything at all costs.
2. **Vegetable oil:** This is some combination of cottonseed, palm, and soybean oil. Note that both the cottonseed and soybean oils

are most likely from genetically modified crops (unless the label says otherwise). And because of the GMO factor alone, I stay away from this greasy goodness (unless organic or certified by the Non-GMO Project) and opt for foods made with other vegetable oils like olive, sunflower, or safflower. Palm is fine; just guard against overconsumption since palm oil is a saturated fat (and its mass production can be harmful to the environment).

3. **Dextrose:** Ah, this is a common sugar euphemism and is all too often added to foods as a sneaky sweetener. While it is not totally offensive, who needs more sugar?

4. **Water:** It is what it is.

5. **Sugar:** It is what it is. But why more? And what is the source— is it sugarcane or the commonly genetically modified sugar beets?

6. **High fructose corn syrup:** Another name for sugar, and one that has made headlines. You've seen not one but three sources of sugar and you are not even halfway through this list of twenty-six substances. Yes, it's important to know where your sugar comes from, but also glance at the grams on your Nutrition Facts Label to keep your pulse on the sugar sum (the Facts definitely come in handy).

7. **Modified food starch (corn and/or wheat):** Starch is a carbohydrate found in plants. It is used as a thickening agent, stabilizer, or emulsifier in food processing. I'll take the starch from the non-GMO corn or unbleached wheat, please. So again, no way of knowing the true source of these ingredients.

8. **Eggs:** This is not an egg as you know it. For processed foods, eggs are typically cracked, pasteurized, and then packaged in either liquid, frozen, or dried form. And I highly doubt they are from hens that were raised humanely.

9. **Nonfat milk:** Again, it is what it is (though it could be powdered), but wouldn't it be lovely if it came from a cow who had a happy life and never had to pop a pill? Doubtful.

10. **Glycerin:** Also called glycerol, glycerin is a sweet, syrupy substance obtained through saponification, the process of adding alkalies (a neutralizing compound) to animal fats (mostly beef) or vegetable oils. Glycerin is a common ingredient in soaps and nitroglycerin (used to create dynamite). So why is it in our food? It is used to promote moisture retention, as in, "I want squishy bread!" I will respectfully decline on glycerin in my food.

11. **Soy flour:** It is what it is, but most likely, you have fallen prey to genetically modified soy again.

12. **Corn syrup solids:** More sugar? You betcha. Corn syrup solids are literally dried corn syrup. And most likely of the GMO variety.

13. **Leavening:** Most commonly known as baking powder or baking soda, these chemical compounds are derived from natural or synthetic sources. Included in the mix is often a starch—typically corn—so yet again, more GMOs.

14. **Preservatives:** This information is so vague that you don't even know what concoctions the manufacturer used to preserve this cracker. This is a red flag for me; chemical preservatives, as defined in the Top-Rated Terminators, just don't fly with me. There are better ways to preserve our food, as you now know.

15. **Salt:** It is what it is.

16. **Natural and artificial flavor:** To recap, both are made in a lab, except the natural flavors are from "natural" sources and the artificial ones from synthetic sources. How about letting food taste like the food itself? But you typically can't when it is highly processed. Manufacturers need to add in flavor to make it suitable and sellable.

17. **Mono- and Diglycerides:** As an emulsifier (keeps oil and water from separating out), these glycerides typically come from partially hydrogenated soybean and canola oil. This is a tough one for me to swallow—trans fats and most likely GMO soy and canola in one shot.

18. **Soy lecithin:** Soy lecithin (in layperson language, fatty substances from soy) is an emulsifier. It also reduces rancidity, reduces spattering in a frying pan, and contributes to the fluffiness of cakes. My only issue is that it most likely comes from GMO soy.

19. **Spices:** It is what it is. No real worries here, other than the possible irradiation factor (as discussed in chapter 1); spices are exposed to radiation to kill off "harmful" bacteria and increase shelf life. Personally, I am not a fan of irradiation. We just don't know enough about this process.

20. **Tapioca starch:** Ground from the cassava plant and used to thicken foods, tapioca starch is what it is.

21. **Wheat starch:** Pretty much the same thing as modified food starch, except that it is definitively from wheat. It is used in food processing as a thickening agent, stabilizer, or emulsifier. Nothing to get up in arms about.

22. **Artificial color:** Need I say more?

23. **Cellulose gum:** Typically made from cotton by-products or wood pulp, cellulose gum is used to improve the texture of food. It also acts as a stabilizer and binding agent. Nothing to scream about but surely the cotton was genetically modified.

24. **Guar and karaya gum:** Derived from natural sources (like bushes, trees, seaweed, and bacteria), gums in general are probably safe but poorly tested. They are primarily used as thickening agents and stabilizers in food. You will often find them in low-fat products to "fill the fat" as they are not absorbed by the body. So you get the body in your food without additions to your belly.

25. **Annatto:** Annatto is a natural food coloring obtained from the seeds of a tropical shrub, the achiote tree. While natural, annatto seems to cause adverse reactions such as hives in some. Consume with caution as per the Center for Science in the Public Interest's *Chemical Cuisine*.

26. **Turmeric:** A spice, and an awesomely healthy one with anti-inflammatory properties. But the amount in this cracker is slim to none, and it's most likely irradiated.

Holy guacamole! This product has twenty-six ingredients, many of which are in my Top-Rated Terminators family. Welcome to the world of fabulous food manufacturing. While some of these ingredients are necessary "evils" in highly processed food, you can surely limit or avoid them when in the know. In fact, a cracker can be made with much fewer ingredients, such as whole-grain brown rice and sesame seeds for a simple yet tasty rice cracker. Or if you fancy a Ritz-like cracker, there is Barbara's Bakery Rite Lite Rounds that contain nine ingredients. In other words, there are better options.

But I must add this: While the FDA requires that all ingredients in your food be listed on your label, the agency also notes in the Code of Federal Regulations that incidental additives that are present in your food at insignificant levels and don't have any technical or functional effect in your food are *exempt* from labeling.[4] This includes ingredients that are incorporated into your food as part of another ingredient (not sure what that really means), processing aids (ingredients that are added but then removed, and those that convert to something that would normally be found in your food), and stuff that is added for its technical and functional effect but is only present in insignificant levels in the finished product. And then there are sulfites that don't have to be listed unless present at a level above 10 parts per million in the end product (wait, shouldn't the FDA *require* sulfite labeling no matter the amount, especially given the potentially severe allergic reaction for many?). In other words, ingredients are likely being added to your food and *do not* require labeling. And while some of this stuff may be totally fine, some may not (like the TRTs). But you really have no way of knowing.

What the Fork to Do

1. The longer the ingredient list, the more processed the food; the shorter the list, the less processed (I generally stick to packaged products with no more than five to seven ingredients).

2. All ingredients lists are written in descending order, meaning that the first ingredient listed is present in the highest quantity in the product. So try to avoid products with sugar as one of the top three to five ingredients.

3. Scrutinize sugar, as it is often present in high quantity in packaged foods and is not just listed as such but also as its many other names and iterations as noted in chapter 5, "Sugar and Its Many Euphemisms."

4. Never trust the word "natural" on a label, as there are no stringent regulations on the real meaning of the word (more on this in sidebar, "'Natural'—Food Labeling Misbehavior to the Max," page 133). While the U.S. government is busy trying to figure out how to define the term in a way that ultimately keeps Big Food content, be super wary of any food product boasting realness.

5. When you see tons of vitamins and minerals on an ingredient list, note that they are added into your foods during processing because the processing of the food strips many of these critical nutrients away.

6. If you can't pronounce it, you probably shouldn't consume it.

7. If you have any food allergies, call the manufacturer directly to inquire about those *insignificant ingredients*.

8. If you want to know specifics about foods and their ingredients including nutritional, health, and environmental implications, check out the Environmental Working Group's Food Database™— the authority for consumer-friendly food transparency at your fingertips. Visit their website at ewg.org for the Food Database™ or download the smartphone app of the same name.

Food Product Claims

In 2012, a popular pomegranate juice beverage was nailed by the Federal Trade Commission (FTC)—the government agency whose mission is to ensure that companies provide truthful information to consumers—for making false claims that it promotes healthy blood vessels, reduces high blood pressure, reduces LDL cholesterol, treats prostate cancer, and alleviates erectile dysfunction. That's professing quite a bit of power in a bottle.

Overhyped claims are epidemic among food products, and I beg you to stop buying into the baloney—like the cookie that touts as much calcium as a glass of milk, as much fiber as a bowl of oatmeal, and as much vitamin C as a bowl of blueberries. Do you *really* think that a cookie is the way to deliver honest nourishment to your precious body? So stop getting duped by "food"; the real deal, as in fresh, whole food, is the way to go.

Whole Foods Defined

According to Annemarie Colbin, PhD, internationally recognized pioneer in the field of whole-foods nutrition, author, speaker, and founder of the Natural Gourmet Institute in New York City, the leader in health-supportive culinary arts and theory (and my alma mater), "whole foods of vegetable origin include fresh vegetables and fruits; whole grains; beans and legumes; nuts and seeds. Whole foods of animal origin include eggs, small whole fish, seafood and small fowl. Under this model, when consuming larger animals (pork, beef, venison) the idea is to use as many parts as possible (muscle, kidney, heart, etc.), including the bones to make stock, to maximize nutrient intake. Eating whole foods ensures consumption of the maximum amount of original natural nutrients, in the right proportions. Conversely, fragmented foods include all foods that are missing original parts."[5] In other words, any food that has been processed to break down or remove pieces is not whole. According to Colbin, a healthy regime is a diet composed of 70 to 80 percent whole foods. It's okay if you are nowhere near that, but how about aiming to get a little closer to that number?

One of my favorite assertions is a sports drink that claims to have "more potassium than five ordinary sports drinks," meaning roughly 250 milligrams. Do we really need this much potassium in a drink? According to the National Institutes of Health's Office of Dietary Supplements, the Recommended Dietary Allowance (RDA)—the average daily intake level sufficient to meet the nutrient requirements of nearly all healthy people—is roughly 3,500 milligrams (mg) per day of potassium. Most Americans can get more than enough from real food like greens including spinach and Swiss chard (about 1,000 mg per 1 cup cooked), white potatoes and yams (about 900 mg per potato), soybeans (about 900 mg per cup), lentils (about 750 mg per cup cooked), avocado (about 700 mg per cup), and banana (about 400 mg each), plus many more whole foods. So why turn to a sugary beverage for any nutrition even if it boasts a bounty of health?

But it doesn't stop there with this "body-protecting" beverage. It also has the "antioxidant equivalent of 1–2 cups of green tea." Guess what? Antioxidants are in practically every whole fresh food, so why get them from a beverage? "More vitamins than a serving of blueberries." The only vitamin to write home about in blueberries is vitamin C, and most likely the C in this beverage is not from blueberries, but added C with blueberry flavor. "Superior nutrition and hydration." Superior to what? A plain old bottle of potassium-rich coconut water with a side of real blueberries and apricots?

Just to be clear, I don't have a problem with functional foods (those that have potentially positive health benefits beyond basic nutrition) by any measure, but what I do have an issue with is the cacophony of claims on highly processed food—because most of the time they are either misleading or just a bunch of empty promises.

To clarify claims, we can break them down into three categories as per the FDA (yes, this agency is also responsible for regulating food promises):

1. *Health claims* characterize the relationship between an ingredient and its ability to reduce the risk of a disease or health-related conditions. For example, "The consumption of omega-3 fatty acids may reduce the risk of coronary heart disease."
2. *Nutrient content claims* characterize the level of a nutrient in the food. Examples include "low-fat," "high fiber," and "only 100 calories."
3. *Structure/function claims* describe the effect a substance has on the structure or function of the body and *do not* make reference to a disease, such as "Calcium builds strong bones."

For most of you, the claims play a critical role in whether or not you grab for a product. But keep this in mind (you are going to love this)—while the FDA regulates these *truthful, non-misleading dietary guidance statements* on food labels, food products *are not reviewed* by the FDA before landing on your grocery store shelf. However, once the food is marketed with a claim, the FDA can consider whether the statement meets the requirement of being truthful and not misleading.

So back to that good old pomegranate juice—the company was sued because the Federal Trade Commission (FTC), a consumer product watchdog, alleged that the company violated federal law by making unsubstantiated claims. The FTC said the studies the company used for evidence were unreliable and not conducted scientifically. Well, the Prince of Pomegranate begged to differ as the corporation spent $35 million to support the scientific research on *their very own products*. I don't know about you, but I think that sounds pretty biased.

To give you an idea of what claims can look like on your food, take a peek at this infamous package to check out some serious claim misbehavior.

Let me help you make sense of this. Do you really think that a highly processed cereal can offer your child immune support? Rely on whole grains, fruits, and vegetables for that purpose. What about the claim that the cereal contains 25 percent of the Daily Value of antioxidants and nutrients? Keep in mind that when a food is highly processed (like cereal), it is stripped of a large percentage of its original vitamins and minerals so what you are getting in your bowl of crunch is either enriched with these micronutrients (added back into food to replace what was lost during processing) or fortified, meaning that

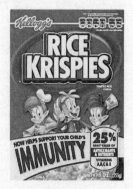

they are simply added to a food "in addition to" rather than to "replace." Typically the nutrients are added back into food in either a powder or liquid form, and are often sprayed on. According to Melanie Warner, nationally recognized journalist and author of *Pandora's Lunchbox*, most of these nutrients don't come from food but originate in a lab from nonfood items; for example, vitamin D can be extracted from the grease in sheep's wool.[6] WTF?

By the way, Kellogg's had to pay $5 million in 2011 to consumers to settle a misleading labeling case brought against them in 2010 by the FTC (Rice Krispies *do not* boost children's immunity). Folks, labels aren't going to stop lying, but hopefully your capacity to fall prey to them will.

What the Fork to Do

1. Generally speaking, don't give too much credence to any claims on processed food, as most likely they are overhyped.
2. A product boasting lots of claims can be a dead giveaway that the food is way too phony.
3. Always know that *real* food, including some products made with five to seven ingredients at most (meaning it is likely not too processed), doesn't need to boast health because more often than not it is *healthy*.

Decoding Food Marketing Madness: The Funny (and Not-So-Funny) Label Lingo

Sadly, because you can't truly trust your food, many other labels have popped up on packages to attempt to better define your edibles—I call this *Funny (and Not-So-Funny) Label Lingo.*

Understanding food labels beyond the Nutrition Facts, ingredient lists, and health claims is critical to making truly healthy choices. In other words, what do terms like "cage-free," "fair trade," "free-range," "grassfed," "hormone-free," "natural," and "organic" really mean for anything plant and animal? And that's just the tip of the iceberg—so trust me when I say that this is the real minefield. The artful terminology used on food and food products is mostly unregulated, but you wouldn't know because it sounds super convincing. Thus, understanding the lingo landscape is part of the battle (like you don't have enough to fight through with food already).

After researching many food labeling guides, I have settled on Animal Welfare Approved's *Food Labels Exposed* (available online at animalwelfareapproved.org or as a smartphone app so you have food guidance at your fingertips) as the most comprehensive and credible source for understanding the language of labels. The *What the Fork* version is what you will see here, and hopefully it will help you determine what to clean out of your pantry, fridge, and freezer and give you the tools to navigate what to buy in the store or, perhaps more importantly, what *not* to buy.

Before getting started, please note that there are terms, like "grassfed," with legal definitions compliments of U.S. food regulating agencies, but there are others lacking legality. In addition, some of the terms are verified (or certified) by an independent third party (a good thing), meaning that a nonbiased auditor ensures that all standards are being met, guaranteeing truth in labeling. To the contrary, many labels are unverified; in other words, no one is looking over these food makers' shoulders (not a good thing) to confirm the honesty of your edibles.

Finally, I have offered suggested directives—as in *"What the Fork* should I do when I see this seal or phrase on my food?" Remember, I aim to meet you where you're at, so here's the info (with visuals where they exist), all truthful to the best of my knowledge, and you decide. By the way, I may have missed some labels, but this is a great start. And, you may see multiple labels and lingo on one package. Understand what each means, then determine their combined truthfulness and insight into actual food transparency.

AMERICAN HUMANE CERTIFIED (AHC)

FOUND ON: Animal edibles

VERIFICATION: Independent third-party verification through AHC

According to the American Humane Association, their more than two hundred science-based welfare standards are based on the internationally recognized "Five Freedoms" developed by the Royal Society for the Prevention of Cruelty to Animals: freedom from hunger or thirst by ready access to fresh water and a diet to maintain full health and vigor; freedom from discomfort by providing an appropriate environment including shelter and a comfortable resting area; freedom from pain, injury, or disease by prevention or rapid diagnosis and treatment; freedom to express normal behavior by providing sufficient space, proper facilities, and company of the animal's own kind; and freedom from fear and distress by ensuring conditions and treatment which avoid mental suffering.[7] But, according to the organization's Standards Guidelines, dairy cattle that live in "fully enclosed housing, artificial lighting must be provided as needed to supplement natural light."[8] In other words, some dairy cattle may never have access to the outdoors. Poultry, which constitute 85 percent of the animals that AHC certifies, live mostly in confinement. The hens live in an enriched colony (giant cages that supposedly give the birds the ability to perch and nest); some are cage-free with *possible* access to the outdoors (AHC certifies 90 percent of all cage-free eggs in the United States); and some are pasture raised. Beak trimming is allowed if deemed necessary (but only prior to 10 days old).[9] Pigs' tails can be docked (or clipped).[10]

DIRECTIVE: If animal welfare (and your health) is ultimately your number one concern, AHC is a step in the right direction but not the ideal—there are certifications with higher humane standards, as you will read shortly.

ANGUS/CERTIFIED ANGUS

FOUND ON: Beef

VERIFICATION: Independent third-party verification through Certified Angus Beef (CAB); if not certified by CAB program, then the label may not be truthful.

The USDA sets forth specific requirements for live cattle to qualify for Angus beef certification programs. Generally speaking: (1) one parent or two registered grandparents must be purebred Angus; or (2) the cattle's appearance must be predominantly (51 percent) black. Once the requirements are met, the beef can be certified by the Certified Angus Beef Program only if ten quality specifications are met in the areas of marbling and maturity, consistent sizing, and quality appearance and tenderness of the beef. According to the website, "The Certified Angus Beef Program was formed in 1978 to provide assurances of beef flavor and tenderness to consumers, who during the 1970s were largely dissatisfied with beef."[11] Note that this seal has nothing to do with how the ruminants are raised, meaning that they are most likely from confined animal feeding operations.

DIRECTIVE: If you care only about the flavor and tenderness of beef, then CAB is for you.

ARTISAN/ARTISANAL

FOUND ON: Cheese, bread, pasta, jams, chocolates, confections, sauces, preserves, condiments, beverages, ice cream, and items from fisheries (and even other products)

VERIFICATION: No

Despite the fact that these terms imply that a product was made by hand and in small batches, anyone can say their product is "artisanal" even if it was factory-produced on a massive scale. At this time, there is no legal definition for these terms and their use is unregulated.

DIRECTIVE: If you want handmade food, best to visit your local farm stand or farmers market. Don't believe mass-produced packaged foods are artisanal.

BIODYNAMIC

FOUND ON: Plant and animal edibles

VERIFICATION: Independent third-party veri- 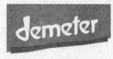 fication; through Demeter; if not certified by Demeter then it may not be truthful

According to the Biodynamic Association, "Biodynamics is a spiritual-ethical-ecological approach to agriculture, food production and nutrition. Biodynamics was first developed in the early 1920s based on the spiritual insights and practical suggestions of the Austrian writer, educator, and social activist Dr. Rudolf Steiner. . . . Biodynamic farmers strive to create a diversified, balanced farm ecosystem that generates health and fertility as much as possible from within the farm itself."[12] The USDA and FDA neither legally define nor regulate biodynamics, but Steiner's definition is widely accepted and respected. The Demeter Association certifies products that meet a stringent set of standards from soil management to raising animals to provide biodynamic assurance to consumers.

DIRECTIVE: If you believe in sustainable agriculture (see page 142 for definition), you can find biodynamic products certified by Demeter, and they fit your budget, definitely buy—a great (if not better) alternative to organic.

CAGE-FREE

FOUND ON: Poultry (though mostly for egg-laying hens) and eggs
VERIFICATION: No

According to the USDA, "[Cage-free] indicates that the flock was able to freely roam a building, room, or enclosed area with unlimited access to food and fresh water during their production cycle."[13] But these birds are often overcrowded and most don't have access to the outdoors. You will often see this label on organics but also on nonorganics.
DIRECTIVE: If you can buy truly cage-free eggs, then it is a step up from meat and eggs from caged birds (though in the end, conditions probably aren't much better). The lack of verification makes this a potentially meaningless term.

CERTIFIED NATURALLY GROWN (CNG)

FOUND ON: Plant and animal edibles, including products from bees
VERIFICATION: No third-party verification but relies on Participatory Guarantee System (PGS) for verification

"Certified Naturally Grown is a grassroots alternative to the USDA's National Organic Program (NOP) meant primarily for small farmers distributing through local channels—farmer's markets, roadside stands, local restaurants, community supported agriculture (CSA) programs and small local grocery stores."[14] CNG was launched in 2002, at the same time the USDA NOP kicked off as an alternative certification for smaller-scale farmers who couldn't manage fees and paperwork requirements of the USDA but were farming organically. Although there is no third-party verification, CNG relies on the Participatory Guarantee System (PGS) for certification—a locally focused quality assurance system based on trust, social networks, and shared knowledge. CNG uses the USDA NOP standards (as you will read shortly) as their foundation, but because they are independent, they can revise and even improve as needed.

DIRECTIVE: If CNG, I would trust that it is organic. CNG truly supports small farms.

CONVENTIONAL

FOUND ON: Plant and animal edibles

VERIFICATION: No (considered the norm)

Simply put, this is the term used to define food that has been grown or raised by standard agricultural practices. It typically includes the use of synthetic fertilizers and pesticides; monocropping (meaning that a farmer grows only one crop versus multiple crops to support biodiversity); genetically modified seeds; concentrated animal feeding operations (CAFOs); and the use of antibiotics and hormones in livestock.

DIRECTIVE: If conventional is all you can do, then it will have to suffice. But hopefully, on some level, you can do better than this as these farming practices do not put your health (or the health of animals and the environment) first. There are plenty of tools in *What the Fork* to push you to do a little better.

COOL (COUNTRY OF ORIGIN LABELING)

FOUND ON: Muscle-cut and ground meats such as beef, veal, pork, lamb, goat, and chicken; wild and farm-raised fish and shellfish; fresh and frozen fruits and vegetables; peanuts, pecans, and macadamia nuts; ginseng

VERIFICATION: No, but the USDA is responsible for enforcing COOL

According to the USDA, COOL is a labeling law that requires

retailers, including chain grocery stores, supermarkets, and club warehouses like BJ's to provide their customers with information about the source of domestic and imported food products (called covered commodities) in *conspicuous* locations (but *not* necessarily on the product itself).[15] COOL has nothing to do with food safety, nor does it offer the consumer any insight into the food "footprint" other than where it originated.

DIRECTIVE: If you want to know where your food came from, then locate the COOL label on or around your covered commodity. If you don't see conspicuous labeling, your retailer is in violation of COOL and you can report them to the COOL director at (202) 720-4486.

FAIR TRADE

FOUND ON: Any nonanimal edible from bananas and dried fruit to cocoa, coffee, and tea

VERIFICATION: Independent third-party verification through several organizations

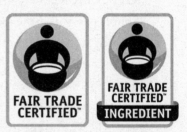

While there is no universally accepted definition for fair trade (it is more of a social movement), several organizations including Fair Trade International, Institute for Market Ecology (IMO), Ecosocial (Brazil), and Fair Trade USA (formerly part of Fair Trade International) have a similar mission: to address the inherent imbalance of power in trading relationships by ensuring better prices, working conditions, local sustainability, and fair terms of trade, ultimately giving the poorest and weakest producers the chance to improve their market position and lives. Several seals denote fair trade including these from Fair Trade USA—products can be 100 percent fair trade (like coffee and other single-ingredient products) or have more than 20 percent fair trade ingredients.

DIRECTIVE: If you can buy anything fair trade, please do so—it's a chance for you to be part of the solution for a more sustainable food system.

FOOD ALLIANCE

FOUND ON: Plant and animal edibles
VERIFICATION: Independent third-party verification through Food Alliance

According to their website, Food Alliance "provides
the food and agriculture industry with sustainability
standards, evaluation tools, and a voluntary, third-party certification
program."[16] The certification is available for more mid-sized family-
scale farms and ranchers, growers, food processors, and distributors,
though they do provide certification for some larger farms. Products
bearing this seal are

- grown by a Food Alliance Certified producer
- packed and/or prepared by a Food Alliance Certified handler
- void of genetically modified crops or livestock
- void of artificial flavors, colors, or preservatives
- humanely cared for (livestock) with no hormones or subtherapeutic
  antibiotics
- traceable through a verified supply chain

In addition, Food Alliance aims to address soil and water conservation, protect biodiversity as well as reduce pesticide use through integrated pest management (a more environmentally friendly way to
manage the chemicals used on food). In addition, they monitor safe and
fair working conditions.

DIRECTIVE: If you see this seal, aim to trust but it does not ensure
organic. For livestock, if you are a stickler like me and want to ensure
that your edible animals were indeed raised on pasture, then don't
hesitate to call the specific Food Alliance Certified producers. Also
Food Alliance has a grassfed certification, as noted on page 127 under
"Grassfed."

FREE-RANGE/FREE-ROAMING

FOUND ON: Animal edibles

VERIFICATION: No

According to the USDA, "Producers must demonstrate to the Agency that poultry has been allowed access to the outside."[17] According to Animal Welfare Approved (one of two organizations with the highest animal welfare standards, as noted under "Humane/High Welfare"), you will never really know if the poultry is roaming in pasture or a dirt lot, or the duration of access to the outdoors, so "free-range" and "free-roaming" are loose terms. For animals other than poultry, there is no legal or regulated definition.

DIRECTIVE: If you can buy free-range/free-roaming, then it is a step up from confined animals (though in the end, conditions probably aren't much better). But the lack of verification makes this a potentially meaningless term.

GLUTEN-FREE

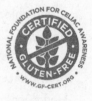

FOUND ON: All packaged edibles

VERIFICATION: Independent third-party verification through the National Foundation for Celiac Awareness (Gluten-Free Certification Program) plus other organizations like the Gluten Intolerance Group (Certified Gluten-Free)

Roughly three million people in the United States have celiac disease— an autoimmune disease whereby gluten damages the absorptive surface of the small intestine, resulting in malabsorption of carbohydrates, fat, protein, vitamins, and minerals and putting them at risk for nutritional deficiencies and other health concerns including osteoporosis, failure to thrive, infertility, miscarriages, and intestinal cancers. According to the FDA, "on August 2, 2013, [the Agency] issued a final rule defining 'gluten-free' for food labeling, which will help consumers, especially those living with celiac disease, be confident that items labeled 'gluten-free' meet a defined standard for gluten content."[18]

DIRECTIVE: If you have celiac disease, feel confident purchasing packaged foods with either seal. Buying certified products is important because all processed food can be exposed to gluten (found in wheat, spelt, kamut, barley, rye, triticale, and oats) during production; verification provides added trust and confidence for those who must be gluten-free.

GMO-FREE

FOUND ON: Plant and seafood edibles

VERIFICATION: Independent third-party verification through the Non-GMO Project

As you now know, genetically modified organisms (GMOs) are plants and animals whose genetics have been altered to give them traits that they would not normally have. Currently there is no *mandatory* labeling for GMOs on any food today, meaning that there is absolutely *no way* for you to know *What the Fork* you are eating. According to the Non-GMO Project, the organization committed to building the non-GMO food supply to offer some level of GMO transparency, "Unfortunately, 'GMO free' and similar claims are not legally or scientifically defensible due to limitations of testing methodology. In addition, the risk of contamination to seeds, crops, ingredients, and products is too high to reliably claim that a product is 'GMO free.' The Project's claim offers a true statement acknowledging the reality of contamination risk, but assuring the shopper that the product in question is in compliance with the Project's rigorous standards."[19] In other words, GMOs have infiltrated the food system so that even non-GMO verification— whether through the Non-GMO Project, USDA Organic, Certified Naturally Grown (CNG), or Food Alliance (FA) certification—can't truly guarantee that your food is 100 percent GMO-free.

DIRECTIVE: If you want GMO-free foods, your best bet is to aim for organics or products bearing the Non-GMO Project seal and/or CNG and FA certification. If you see "Non-GMO" without the project's seal or any of the others, the claim is not verified.

GRASSFED

FOUND ON: Cattle, sheep, goats, and bison
VERIFICATION: Independent third-party verification through the American Grassfed Association (AGA), Animal Welfare Approved (AWA), and Food Alliance (FA)

According to the USDA, "Grass and forage shall be the feed source consumed for the lifetime of the ruminant animal, with the exception of milk consumed prior to weaning. The diet shall be derived solely from forage consisting of grass (annual and perennial), forbs (e.g., legumes, *Brassica*), browse, or cereal grain crops in the vegetative (pre-grain) state. Animals cannot be fed grain or grain byproducts and must have continuous access to pasture during the growing season."[20] However, "incidental grain supplementation" is permitted without stringent guidelines. In other words, your cattle can be in the USDA grassfed program, can be fed grain and still remain in the program and be sold to you as "grassfed."[21]

The American Grassfed Association (AGA) verifies that not only are the animals truly grassfed as noted here, but also that they are truly raised on pasture (versus having "access to pasture") without any confinement and never given drugs. AWA and FA do the same. While AWA and FA don't necessarily have separate seals for "grassfed" you may note the terminology on or near their existing labels.

Also AGA suggests that "grass finished" is a marketing claim with no legal definition. While it implies that animals are grassfed at some point in their lives, it's for an undefined period. The term does not indicate whether the animal was raised in confinement or given drugs.[22]

DIRECTIVE: If you want truly grassfed animal foods trust AGA as well as AWA and FA. As for grass-finished, this term is loosely defined and does not mean that animals were exclusively grassfed.

HEIRLOOM

FOUND ON: Plant edibles
VERIFICATION: No
While no legal definition exists, heirlooms represent unique plant varieties (maintained though crop cultivation, selection, and seed saving) that are distinct from their commercial counterparts commonly found in industrialized agriculture. This term has nothing to do with farming practices.
DIRECTIVE: If you can find heirlooms, give them a try for some variety. But note that just because your plant is unique, there is no guarantee that it was grown without chemicals unless USDA Organic or Certified Naturally Grown.

HERITAGE

FOUND ON: Animal edibles
VERIFICATION: No
According to the Livestock Conservancy, "heritage" ensures genetic conservation and promotion of endangered breeds of livestock and poultry that are part of U.S. agricultural history.[23] However, the label is not officially recognized by the USDA; neither is the term "policed."
DIRECTIVE: If you see *heritage*, don't automatically assume good health—this term has nothing to do with how your animals were raised. As there is no verification, the term is loosely used on animal foods. If you want to understand specifics about a product's heritage, contact the producer to learn more.

HUMANE/HIGH WELFARE

FOUND ON: Animal edibles
VERIFICATION: Independent third-party verification through Animal Welfare Approved and Certified Humane Raised and Handled
DIRECTIVE: Although there is no formal definition for humane/high welfare, and you should be super cautious about producers making

such claims, two organizations stand out for offering highly transparent and credible independent third-party certifications for farmers.

ANIMAL WELFARE APPROVED (AWA)

A national nonprofit, AWA audits, certifies, and supports family farms that put the animal at the center of the system. There are specific standards for every farm animal, from cattle and hens to the dogs that work the farm. Creatures live on pasture without confinement, are fed the diet they were meant to eat (for example, cows eat grass), and are never given drugs subtherapeutically. High-welfare slaughter practices are a must, meaning the animals are loved to the last minute (believe it or not, this is possible).

CERTIFIED HUMANE RAISED AND HANDLED

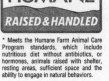

Commonly referred to as Certified Humane, this verification is comparable to AWA and is dedicated to "improving the lives of farm animals in food production from birth to slaughter."[24] They have a highly stringent set of standards that producers must meet for their end products to bear the Certified Humane seal.

To learn more about the difference in animal welfare ratings, check out certifiedhumane.org/standardscomparisonchart.pdf.

According to AWA and Certified Humane, animals are treated with drugs only to reduce pain and suffering; drugs are administered responsibly and judiciously.

DIRECTIVE: If you see a product with AWA or Certified Humane, then you can trust that you are getting the healthiest animal edible for you and the environment. While products are not yet widely available in stores, you can find them through both organizations' websites (animalwelfareapproved.org and certifiedhumane.org).

IRRADIATION

FOUND ON: Fresh fruits and vegetables, lettuce and spinach, spices and seasonings; seeds for sprouting (like alfalfa sprouts); as well as beef, pork, poultry, shellfish, and fresh shell eggs

VERIFICATION: No, but regulated by FDA for non-animal foods and the USDA for animal foods

Food irradiation is a technology for controlling spoilage and eliminating food-borne pathogens on animal and plant foods. Three sources of radiation approved for use on food are gamma rays, X-rays, and electron beam (or e-beam). According to the FDA, "irradiated foods [must] bear the international symbol for irradiation. Look for the radura symbol along with the statement 'Treated with radiation' or 'Treated by irradiation' on the food label. Bulk foods, such as fruits and vegetables, are required to be individually labeled or to have a label next to the sale container. FDA does not require that individual ingredients in multi-ingredient foods (e.g., spices) be labeled."[25]

DIRECTIVE: If you want to avoid irradiated foods, keep an eye out for the radura and/or "Treated with radiation" or "Treated by irradiation."

KOSHER

FOUND ON: Animal and plant edibles

VERIFICATION: Independent third-party verification through OU Kosher

OU (Orthodox Union) Kosher, the most trusted global certifier, states that "kosher laws have their origin in the Bible, and are detailed in the Talmud and the other codes of Jewish traditions."[26] According to OU, "the Bible lists the basic categories of food items which are not kosher. These include certain animals, fowl and fish (such as pork and rabbit, eagle and owl, catfish and sturgeon), most insects, and any shellfish or reptile. In addition, kosher species of meat and fowl must be slaughtered in a prescribed manner, and meat and dairy products may not be manufactured or consumed together." The USDA allows "Kosher" on labels of meat and poultry products prepared under rabbinical supervision.

DIRECTIVE: If you keep kosher, then let OU certification guide you. It has nothing do to with organics or animal welfare.

LOCALLY GROWN

FOUND ON: Plant and animal edibles
VERIFICATION: No

According to the USDA, "there is no consensus on a definition of 'local' or 'local food systems' in terms of the geographic distance between production and consumption. But defining 'local' based on marketing arrangements, such as farmers selling directly to consumers at regional farmers' markets or to schools, is well recognized."[27] The USDA notes that the term is used to describe a more localized method of food production and distribution rather than the commonplace national and international industrialized system.

DIRECTIVE: If you can buy local, it is definitely the way to go. Local organic is ideal, but if you can't find that, I encourage you to consume what's closest to home even if with chemicals. Supporting the local farmer is central to rebuilding local economies.

NATURAL

FOUND ON: Anything edible whatsoever (even body care and household products)
VERIFICATION: No

Currently, the FDA has *not* developed a formal definition for the term "natural;" however, according to the agency, they have not objected to its use on "food that does not contain added color, artificial flavors or synthetic substances."[28]

According to the USDA, "meat, poultry, and egg products labeled as 'natural' must be minimally processed and contain no artificial ingredients. However, the natural label does not include any standards regarding farm practices and only applies to processing of meat and egg products. There are no standards or regulations for the labeling of natural food products if they do not contain meat or eggs."[29]

DIRECTIVE: If a product claims to be "natural," please beware. It is a misused and overused term (see the following sidebar, "'Natural'— Food Labeling Misbehavior to the Max").

"Natural"—Food Labeling Misbehavior to the Max

Have you ever seen *The Natural Effect*? This video educates consumers about the artful use and abuse of the term "natural" by the food industry. Thanks are due to the Organic Trade Association, the membership-based organization that focuses on organic trade in North America, for its efforts to begin building a necessary barricade for the baloney.

In March 2013, the FDA had this to say about *natural*, a term that you now know is loosely defined: "From a food science perspective, it is difficult to define a food product that is 'natural' because the food has probably been processed and is no longer the product of the earth. That said, [the] FDA has not developed a definition for use of the term natural or its derivatives. However, the agency has not objected to the use of the term if the food does not contain added color, artificial flavors, or synthetic substances."[30]

I know it may seem confusing. You see the term "natural" or "naturally" on the package, possibly a picture of a farm or meadow, and you are convinced. But in reality, *natural* means nothing anymore, as its overuse and misuse has utterly adulterated what it once represented decades ago—food that was truly pure (made with few ingredients, meaning not too processed; void of anything utterly inventive like flavors made in a lab; and GMO-free).

This term is too loosely defined, giving the food industry the advantage of labeling anything they want as *natural* and duping you into believing that you are doing the right thing. Folks, an overly ranchified bag of chips, having ten to fifteen ingredients, including "natural" flavors (their source being natural rather than synthetic) and genetically modified favorites such as corn, soy, and cottonseed oil, is not natural.

Proponents of grassroots organic and USDA Organic (among many other food watchdogs) are fighting to salvage food integrity by pleading with the FDA to rethink this nonsense term and give it the definition it deserves, particularly ensuring that it should never coexist with genetically modified organisms in any way.

But this is the deal—the Grocery Manufacturers Association (GMA), the multibillion-dollar lobbying group that supports junk food manufacturers, pesticide companies, and Big Pharma, begs to differ. As individual states continue to fight for their Right to Know GMOs pleading for *mandatory* labeling, the GMA is trying to coerce the FDA with their Coalition for Safe and Affordable Food to create a *voluntary* GMO labeling law. Hmmm . . .

What does that mean? According to Organic Consumers Association, a public-interest NGO campaigning for health, justice, and sustainability (and another of my go-to food and environment watchdogs), "Companies that pollute your environment and poison your food want the FDA to come up with a worthless, voluntary labeling standard. And oh by the way, they also want the FDA to rule that it's perfectly fine to label GMO-contaminated food as 'natural.'"[31]

Your best bet to make a difference is to scrutinize anything claiming to be "natural," take action through any of the Food Policy, Safety, and Accountability organizations in Appendix E, "Redeemable Resources." And let the FDA know what you think by calling 1-888-SAFEFOOD.

NATURALLY RAISED

FOUND ON: Animal edibles

VERIFICATION: No

In 2009, the USDA issued a voluntary standard for "naturally raised" livestock. According to the department, "[naturally raised] livestock used for the production of meat and meat products have been raised entirely without growth promotants [or] antibiotics, and have never been fed animal by-products."[32]

DIRECTIVE: If you can buy naturally raised, then it is a step up from animals given drugs. But the lack of verification makes this a potentially meaningless term.

NO ADDITIVES

FOUND ON: Plant and animal edibles

VERIFICATION: No

The FDA defines a food additive as "any substance added to food. Legally, the term refers to 'any substance the intended use of which results or may reasonably be expected to result—directly or indirectly—in its becoming a component or otherwise affecting the characteristics of any food. This definition includes any substance used in the production, processing, treatment, packaging, transportation or storage of food. The purpose of the legal definition, however, is to impose a premarket approval requirement. Therefore, this definition excludes ingredients whose use is generally recognized as safe [GRAS] (where government approval is not needed), those ingredients approved for use by FDA or the [USDA] prior to the food additives provisions of law, and color additives and pesticides where other legal premarket approval requirements apply."[33] While food additives need preapproval, items that are GRAS do not. So technically this term is loosely defined.

DIRECTIVE: If your food says "no additives," check your ingredient lists to investigate. While there technically may be "no additives," there may be plenty of GRAS substances (remember, they are not considered "additives" by the FDA).

NO ANIMAL BY-PRODUCTS

FOUND ON: Animal edibles

VERIFICATION: No

According to Animal Welfare Approved (AWA), "Animal by-products are the parts of a slaughtered animal that are not directly consumed by humans. This includes fat, bones and gelatin. The vast majority of this material is 'rendered' or processed to produce a ground meal called meat and bone meal, which is used in the formulation of animal feed to improve protein levels." Fish meal is also commonly used in livestock feed. According to AWA, "scientists have linked a number of major animal disease outbreaks to the feeding of animal by-products to farm animals."[34] This is good for neither the animal nor you. In 2008, the FDA issued a feed ban specifying cattle material prohibited in animal feed (CMPAF) in response to concerns over mad cow disease (bovine spongiform encephalopathy, BSE), a fatal neurodegenerative disease found in cattle and transferrable to humans if contaminated meat is consumed. Thus, BSE-positive cattle as well as parts of the carcass most commonly infected with BSE (brain, spinal cord, digestive tract, and tallow) are no longer allowed in livestock feed. But other animal parts not specified as CMPAF are still permitted (though cows are never fed cows).

DIRECTIVE: If you can buy animal food with "no animal by-products," then it's a step up from the norm. But the lack of verification makes this a potentially meaningless term.

NO ANTIBIOTICS

FOUND ON: Animal edibles (including dairy and eggs)
VERIFICATION: No

According to the USDA, "'no antibiotics added' may be used on labels for meat or poultry products if sufficient documentation is provided by the producer to the Agency demonstrating that the animals were raised without antibiotics."[35]

DIRECTIVE: If you can buy animal food with "no antibiotics," then it's a step up from the norm. But the lack of verification makes this a potentially meaningless term.

NO HORMONES ADDED/ADMINISTERED

FOUND ON: Beef (including dairy)

VERIFICATION: No

According to the USDA, "hormones are not allowed in raising hogs or poultry. Therefore, the claim 'no hormones added' cannot be used on the labels of pork or poultry unless it is followed by a statement that says 'Federal regulations prohibit the use of hormones.'"

For beef, "no hormones administered" may be approved for use on the label, according to the USDA, "if sufficient documentation is provided to the Agency by the producer showing no hormones have been used in raising the animals."[36]

DIRECTIVE: If you can buy animal food with "no hormones added/administered," then it's a step up from the norm. But the lack of verification makes this a potentially meaningless term.

NO NITRATES/NITRITES

FOUND ON: Lunch meats, hot dogs, bacon, and cured meats

VERIFICATION: No

The addition of nitrates/nitrites has been controversial for years because of their association with increased risk of cancer. According to the EPA, "exposure to higher levels of nitrates or nitrites has been associated with increased incidence of cancer in adults, and possible increased incidence of brain tumors, leukemia, and nasopharyngeal (nose and throat) tumors in children in some studies but not others. Thus the U.S. EPA concluded that there was conflicting evidence in the literature as to whether exposures to nitrate or nitrites are associated with cancer in adults and in children."[37] So they are still allowed in food, but several producers have voluntarily stopped using the chemicals. When you see "no nitrates/nitrites" in meats, it means that the synthetics were not added as a preservative. But celery powder and celery juice, both of which contain *naturally occurring* nitrates and nitrites, are often used to preserve the color of meats.

DIRECTIVE: If you have to use these meats, go with the "free" version, but consume these curious foods minimally. This term relates only to how the item was processed.

NO SPRAY/PESTICIDE-FREE

FOUND ON: Plant edibles

VERIFICATION: No

You may see this term on nonorganic produce labels that want to boast that they are not sprayed with chemicals.

DIRECTIVE: If you want pesticide-free (or semi-pesticide-free) produce, aim for USDA Organic, biodynamic, or Certified Naturally Grown. It is the only way to hopefully ensure that your plants were not sprayed with offensive chemicals.

OMEGA-3 ENRICHED

FOUND ON: Eggs

VERIFICATION: No

Hens are fed omega-3-rich flax to make their eggs "healthier" for you. However, hens (as well as cattle) raised on pasture are naturally rich in omega-3 fats without dietary additions.

DIRECTIVE: If you want to spend a little extra money on eggs for this "added value," then go ahead. And don't forget that truly pasture-raised eggs are inherently rich in the omegas so I suggest putting your dollars here.

ORGANIC (USDA CERTIFIED)

FOUND ON: All things edible (excluding fish)

VERIFICATION: Independent third-party verification through the USDA National Organic Program

According to the USDA National Organic Program (NOP), "*organic* is a labeling term indicating that a food or other agricultural product integrates cultural, biological, and mechanical

practices that foster cycling of resources, promotes ecological balance, and conserves biodiversity. Synthetic fertilizers, sewage sludge, irradiation, and genetic engineering are not permitted."[38] For plants, the organic seal "verifies that irradiation, sewage sludge, synthetic fertilizers, prohibited pesticides [certain NOP-approved chemicals are allowed to be used in organic farming and processing], and genetically modified organisms were not used."[39] For animals, it "verifies that producers met animal health and welfare standards, did not use antibiotics or growth hormones, used 100% organic feed, and provided animals with access to the outdoors."[40] And for foods with multiple ingredients, the seal "verifies that the product has 95% or more certified organic content." Do note that products with less than 95 percent organic ingredients cannot bear the seal. There is also a "made with organic" label that has at least 70 percent organic content, and the rest of the nonorganic ingredients are not allowed to contain GMOs.

DIRECTIVE: If you can buy organic across the board or even partially, I urge you to do so.* While USDA NOP does approve some pesticides for use, the list is limited and much better than conventional practices. For animal edibles, the seal does not necessarily mean that your animals were fed their ideal (as in grass for cattle) or that they have sufficient access to the outdoors (as in raised on pasture). As the use of any drugs is prohibited, if an animal gets sick and needs antibiotics, it is removed from the organic program. Animal foods that bear the USDA Organic seal with additional Animal Welfare Approved or Certified Humane verifications could very well be the closest thing to ideal.

PASTURED/PASTURE RAISED

FOUND ON: Animal edibles

VERIFICATION: No

---

*While organic is not necessarily *more nutritious* than nonorganic according to that 2012 Stanford University Study,[41] the organic advantage is the minimal detectable pesticide residues (7 percent), while their conventional counterparts showed a 38 percent presence. So let's see organic for what it really is—an overall healthier choice for you and the environment (including a non-GMO "guarantee"), and that's good enough for me.

According to the USDA, "Due to the number of variables involved in pasture-raised agricultural systems, the USDA has not developed a federal definition for pasture-raised products."[42]

So, if you see this term on your food label, unless it is certified by Animal Welfare Approved, you have no way of knowing if your animal was truly raised on a pasture.

DIRECTIVE: If you can buy animal food with "Pastured/Pasture-Raised," then it could be many steps up from the norm. But the lack of verification makes this a potentially meaningless term.

RAINFOREST ALLIANCE CERTIFIED

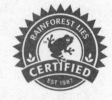

FOUND ON: Products including cocoa, coffee and fruit

VERIFICATION: Third-party verification through the Rainforest Alliance; certification is awarded to farms that meet the comprehensive criteria of the Sustainable Agriculture Network (SAN)

Companies that source products from Rainforest Alliance Certified farms may feature the little green frog seal, indication that the product—or a main ingredient contained in the product—was grown and harvested in accordance with a set of very high standards relating to environmental, social, and economic sustainability. The comprehensive program gives producers the knowledge and skills to manage their farms using methods that encompass all aspects of sustainability and empower them to negotiate the global marketplace themselves. According to the Rainforest Alliance, "farmers engaged in the Rainforest Alliance Certified program learn to grow smart, increasing their bottom line today, and conserving the fertile soils and natural resources on which their children will depend tomorrow."[43]

DIRECTIVE: If you can Shop the Frog, I urge you to do so. Check out rainforest-alliance.org/green-living/shopthefrog to learn more.

RAW

FOUND ON: Dairy including milk, milk products, and cheese
VERIFICATION: No

You've probably heard about it and seen it on some packages. Because of a high incidence of food-borne illness, many food items including milk, cheese, and other dairy products are pasteurized (heat-treated) to ward off pathogens. When a product says *raw*, it means that it was not pasteurized. There is no legal or regulated definition.

DIRECTIVE: If you want to consume raw dairy, please do so with caution (however, pregnant women and children should avoid it). While the FDA believes that raw dairy can pose serious health risks because of the presence of dangerous microorganisms, some health experts believe it has superior nutrition.

rBGH-FREE

FOUND ON: Dairy including milk, milk products, and cheese
VERIFICATION: No

Genetically engineered recombinant bovine growth hormone (rBGH), created by Monsanto, are given to cows to boost milk production. According to Food and Water Watch, not only do these hormones negatively impact the animals' health, but also some studies suggest that use of these drugs can put human health at risk by altering hormone levels in people. While dairy products such as milk and cheese can boast this claim, there is no legal definition and it is not regulated.

DIRECTIVE: If you can buy rBGH-free dairy, then it's a step up from the norm. But the lack of verification makes this a potentially meaningless term.

SULFITE-FREE/NO ADDED SULFITES/CONTAINS SULFITES

FOUND ON: Condiments and relishes; sugar derived from sugar beets; molasses; fresh or frozen shrimp and lobster; canned clams; gelatins, puddings, and fillers; jams and jellies; shredded coconut; processed vegetables (canned, pickled, instant, or frozen); dried soup mixes; syrups including corn and maple; and instant tea and alcoholic beverages including beer, wine, wine coolers, and mixers

VERIFICATION: No

Sulfites are added to foods for preservation. And they can cause an allergic reaction in many. In wine production, sulfites can be added but they also occur naturally as part of the fermentation process. A wine is "sulfite-free" if there are no detectable sulfites when tested. "No added sulfites" means that the sulfites are naturally occurring. And as it relates to wine and other foods, "contains sulfites," whether added or naturally occurring, means that the sulfite-to-food ratio is at or above ten parts per million.

DIRECTIVE: If you have a sulfite sensitivity or allergy, be hypervigilant about understanding this claim, as there is no formal verification. Issues with sulfites should not be taken lightly, so I urge you to contact food producers to understand potential content in suspect foods, as labeling can be inconsistent.

SUSTAINABLE AGRICULTURE

FOUND ON: Anything edible

VERIFICATION: No

As written in the 1990 Farm Bill, "the term sustainable agriculture means an integrated system of plant and animal production practices having a site-specific application that will, over the long term:

- Satisfy human food and fiber needs
- Enhance environmental quality and the natural resource base upon which the agricultural economy depends
- Make the most efficient use of nonrenewable resources and on-farm resources and integrate, where appropriate, natural biological cycles and controls

- Sustain the economic viability of farm operations
- Enhance the quality of life for farmers and society as a whole."

DIRECTIVE: If you can buy from producers who are sustainably farming, then you are making a real difference not only in the health of the producers, plants, animals, your local community, and the environment, but also in your own health. But the lack of verification makes this a potentially meaningless term. However, many certifications noted in this section promote and verify sustainable practices.

TRANSITIONAL

FOUND ON: Plant edibles
VERIFICATION: No

If you shop at Whole Foods, you may see such signage on piles of produce. It means that the farm growing your food is in the midst of transitioning to organic farming practices. But before it can become a certified organic farm, it must practice three years of organic farming.

DIRECTIVE: If you can buy "transitional," then it's a step up from the norm. But the lack of verification makes this a potentially meaningless term.

VEGETARIAN-FED/FED A VEGETARIAN DIET

FOUND ON: Animal edibles
VERIFICATION: No

This label suggests that your animal was fed a vegetarian diet, as in "no animal by-products." It doesn't say anything about the way your animal was raised, like whether it had pasture access or was regularly administered drugs.

DIRECTIVE: If you can buy "Vegetarian-Fed/Fed a Vegetarian Diet," then it's a step up from the norm. But the lack of verification makes this a potentially meaningless term.

WHOLE GRAIN

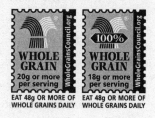

FOUND ON: Grain-based products

VERIFICATION: Independent third-party verification through the Whole Grains Council

This is a great tool to help you navigate products that are indeed made with whole grains, but this seal can appear on a cookie just as well as on a bag of steel-cut oats. According to the Whole Grains Council, "Consumers searching the grocery aisles for authentic whole grain foods now have an effective 'search tool'—the Whole Grain Stamp."[44] The council notes that a whole grain is the entire seed (or kernel) of certain grasses, containing all three of its original edible parts: the bran, germ, and endosperm. All three parts deliver valuable nutrition to a food. On the seal, there are two variations: "100% whole grain" means that all grain ingredients in the product are indeed whole; and the basic stamp ensures that the product contains at least 8 grams of whole grains per serving (but it may also contain some refined grain).

DIRECTIVE: Definitely go for edibles with this seal, but be sure to choose wisely and don't forget that intact whole grains—like brown rice, oats, or quinoa—with little or no processing are still healthiest.

For a more comprehensive list of food labels and their definitions, visit animalwelfareapproved.org/food-labels-exposed/.

What the Fork to Do

You may be thinking that matters just got worse. How the heck are you supposed to navigate food with all the facts, ingredients, claims, and now these other noshing nuances—*What the Fork*! But a little advice: You now have just a bit more consumption clarity, giving you more tools to ask some necessary questions about your food. If it's of any comfort, even knowing all that I do, my head is spinning. So how do you take the information packed in these pages and apply it? First, here is a list of the lingo that I rely on to tell the story of my food:

1. Biodynamic
2. Certified Naturally Grown (CNG)
3. Fair trade
4. Food Alliance Certified (using discretion)
5. GMO-free whether organic or certified by the Non-GMO Project
6. Grassfed as certified by the American Grassfed Association (AGA), Animal Welfare Approved (AWA) or Food Alliance (FA)
7. Humane/high-welfare as certified by Animal Welfare Approved (AWA) and Certified Humane
8. Locally grown
9. Organic (USDA)
10. Rainforest Alliance Certified
11. Whole grain as certified by Whole Grains Council
12. Terms like "cage-free," "free-roaming," "grassfed," "no antibiotics," "no hormones," "no animal by-products," "naturally raised," "no rBGH," "pasture raised" and "vegetarian-fed" have meaning to me only if the food is also labeled USDA Organic, Biodynamic or CNG with, AGA, AWA and/or Certified Humane and FA labels to boot (this the ideal that I aim for most of the time).

And now it's time for you to decide what works for you and what doesn't. Know that this shift will not happen overnight, and baby steps are perfectly fine. What you decide often depends on where you are, what is available, and, of course, the money in your pocket. My goal is to meet you where you're at but push you just a tad to do a little better. So I simply urge you to learn thy labels and use them as tools as you pilot products.

You have officially completed Food Labels 101. Congratulations! Now is it time to apply this knowledge in your DIY Pantry, Fridge, and Freezer Rehab.

Food Fraud

Your food is experiencing an identity crisis. Wrongful labeling is an ongoing concern. In fact, a 2013 ABC News report on counterfeit food revealed some startling findings from the U.S. Pharmacopeial (USP) Convention—an NGO whose mission is to improve the health of people globally through public standards that ensure the quality, safety, and benefit of foods (and medicines).[45] Apparently 7 percent of the U.S. food supply contains fraudulent ingredients (up 60 percent from 2011). Tea is cut with lawn grass; spices like black pepper and paprika are filled with starches or other less expensive spices; olive oil is diluted with cheaper stuff like soybean oil; pomegranate juice is not all that—it often contains a little pear and grape juice too; and 100 percent pure lemon juice is often modified with water and sugar. Liquids and ground foods are the main culprits, so you are safer with whole foods like the peppercorn that you grind yourself. But the reality is that everyone consumes some, if not many, impure foods. So what to do?

Sadly, consumers have very little to go on when identifying faux food. The Food and Drug Administration can't test everything. But thanks to USP's Food Fraud Database (usp.org/food/ingredients/food-fraud-database), you can be kept in the loop about fakers. The only caveat is that they don't offer information about specific brands, so in the end, you know tons about what to look out for, but you don't know which companies are deceiving you to ultimately better their bottom line. A bit of advice: Avoid the price cuts and super-size containers of liquids and ground herbs and spices—if the food is cheap, it is more likely to have been adulterated. I know this isn't much information to go on, and it's quite disconcerting to find out that you've probably been eating some phonies, but that makes it all the more reason for you to embrace a little edible skepticism.

CHAPTER 12

Do-It-Yourself (DIY) Pantry, Fridge, and Freezer Rehab

While watching *America's Funniest Home Videos* with my kids, I saw a woman open her pantry to have her brother, dressed as the Grim Reaper, scare the bejesus out of her. It was quite a sight and surely something any number of boys in my life would do to me. As metaphors often move me, please answer this: Does the Grim Reaper live among your food? Let's find out. While I can't stand by your side as you evaluate your pantry, I can absolutely give you the tools you need to get the "bad" out. Four central tasks are involved in this process:

1. Identify the foods containing the Top-Rated Terminators (we will call these the Grim Reapers—dramatic, I know, but you now know I like metaphors).
2. Identify the "safe" foods (we will call these the Keepers).
3. Create a strategy around removing the Grim Reapers and replacing them with the Better for You Alternatives.
4. Determine which unhealthy foods you Can't Live Without (let's call these compromises, something I am all for, as long as you are making well-informed decisions). See sidebar, "Can't Live Without," page 176 to learn all about this.

Be sure to read through chapters 12 and 13 in their entirety before taking any rehab action.

The Pantry

Take a look in your pantry (or cabinets if you don't have a larder of sorts). Do you have that obligatory canister of bread crumbs with hydrogenated oils, tucked behind the cans of soup loaded with MSG? Or perhaps maple syrup that consists of corn syrup and nothing maple other than artificial flavoring? And, while we are on a roll, do you have a bottle of vegetable oil that was opened, used once, and stashed? Turn that top and take a whiff. Does it have a smell? The answer is most likely "Yes," and the smell can probably be likened to that of a mild paint thinner. Folks, your oil is rancid. When was the last time you used it? How about your spices? One of my clients in 2011 had spices that dated back as far as 1995. Are you getting my gist? You literally and figuratively shelve the things you don't want to deal with. And your pantry is suffering. So it's time to psychoanalyze your food.

As we discussed before, the TRTs will forever be controversial among government, Big Food, Big Ag, and the biotech, science, and health communities at large. While there is plenty of evidence to question most, if not all of them, there is not enough to deem them unsafe for human consumption, or to issue a cease-and-desist order. So while some studies can assure you that many of these ingredients are harmless, you definitely know where my bias lies—why take any risk with your health, or more important, that of your little loved ones?

Now that you have the Top-Rated Terminators and Food Labels 101 under your belts, you are ready to pull from your pantry.

TO PREP FOR THE MAKEOVER:

1. Clear your table and countertops to make room for the goods; you will need the space as you pull foods, determine their fate, and organize.

2. Designate an area for the Grim Reapers (the garbage is a good place, although do take a look at the sidebar, "Your Local Food Pantry," below) and the Keepers.
3. Have the Top-Rated Terminator Very Quick Reference Guide (discussed shortly) handy to keep you on your toes with noted ingredients.
4. Have the Environmental Working Group's Food Database[TM]— available online at ewg.org or as a smartphone app—as backup just in case you want more information on specific ingredients. You may just have an appetite for further detail.

Your Local Food Pantry

You may notice that many of your Grim Reapers are unopened. If so, I ask that you to donate them to a local food pantry. While my ideal is to eliminate consumption of all foods containing TRTs, there are people going hungry every day, and any food is better than no food.

If you can, consider making "food giving" a regular thing, aiming to offer true nourishment to those in need—in other words, foods without my TRTs. SuperFood Drive is a global organization whose mission is to relieve hunger through healthy food distribution by way of food banks and food pantries. This healthy hunger-relief initiative provides resources from shopping lists for donors to recipes for recipients as well as education and tools on how to create and provide true nourishment to all. To learn more, check out superfooddrive.org.

TOP-RATED TERMINATOR
VERY QUICK REFERENCE GUIDE

TOP-RATED TERMINATOR	INGREDIENT REFERENCE
Chemical Preservatives	Sodium benzoate or any benzoate; potassium sorbate or any sorbate; potassium bisulfite, potassium metabisulfite, sodium bisulfite, sodium metabisulfite, sodium sulfite; sodium nitrate, sodium nitrite; butylated hydroxyanisole (BHA), butylated hydroxytoluene (BHT); propyl gallate; tert-butylhydroquinone (TBHQ)
Artificial Flavors and Enhancers	Anything that says "artificial flavors" or "flavoring" (even "natural flavors," if you want to take it that far); monosodium glutamate (MSG)
Artificial Colors	Anything that says "artificial colors" or "coloring"; Red Dye No. 40 (red #40); Yellow Dye No. 5 (yellow #5); Yellow Dye No. 6 (yellow #6); any other Dye No. And anything that says "Lake," such as "Blue 1 Lake"
Artificial Sweeteners	Acesulfame-K, acesulfame potassium, ace-K, Sunett, Sweet One; aspartame, NutraSweet, Equal, Sugar Twin; neotame; saccharin, Sweet'N Low, Sweet Twin, Necta Sweet; sucralose, Splenda. Also be mindful of the sugar alcohols and novel sweeteners: erythritol, hydrogenated starch hydrosolates, isomalt, lactitol, maltitol, mannitol, sorbitol, xylitol; stevia, Reb A, PureVia, Truvia; fructo-oligosaccharide (FOS); tagatose, Naturalose; and trehalose

TOP-RATED TERMINATOR	INGREDIENT REFERENCE
Sugar and Its Many Euphemisms	Agave, Barbados sugar, barley malt, beet sugar, brown sugar, buttered syrup, cane juice crystals, cane sugar, caramel, corn syrup, corn syrup solids, confectioner's sugar, carob syrup, castor sugar, date sugar, demerara sugar, dextrin, dextrose, diastatic malt, diatase, Florida crystals, fructose, fruit juice, fruit juice concentrate, galactose, glucose, glucose solids, golden sugar, golden syrup, grape sugar, high-fructose corn syrup, honey, icing sugar, invert sugar, lactose, maltodextrin, malt syrup, maple syrup, molasses, muscovado sugar, panela, raw sugar, refiner's syrup, rice syrup, sorghum syrup, Sucanat, sucrose, sugar, treacle, turbinado sugar, yellow sugar
Trans Fats (Hydrogenated Oils)	Hydrogenated oil, partially hydrogenated oil; shortening; margarine
Chemical Pesticides	This is not something that you will typically see on a label, but note that anything organic is hopefully void of these chemicals; anything partially organic is not, as in "contains organic ingredients"; for produce, check out Pesticides in Produce (aka the Dirty Dozen Plus™ and the Clean 15™) from the Environmental Working Group.
Antibiotics and Hormones	You may see "antibiotic-free" and/or "hormone-free" on labels, but you really need to know how to vet through them, as noted in chapter 11, "Food Labels 101."

TOP-RATED TERMINATOR	INGREDIENT REFERENCE
Genetic Modification	Unless organic, anything with alfalfa, canola, corn, cotton, papaya, soy, and sugar beets is most likely genetically modified. Best bet is to check out the Non-GMO Project's *Shopping Guide* or *True Food* by the Center for Food Safety to get the latest and greatest information (more on this in chapter 14).

On Big Food

Not to be a downer, but if your product is made by one of the super-large food companies like ConAgra, then chances are that the product is not great for your health, since that is not their number-one priority. That being said, some of these companies do have some incredibly decent brands (mostly because they "ate" smaller companies that were doing the right thing). For example, General Mills, notorious for Betty Crocker, also owns two of my most favorite brands, Cascadian Farms (frozen fruits and vegetables) and Muir Glen (canned tomato products); and Kellogg's, creators of Pop-Tarts, owns organic Green & Black's chocolate.

Know this: For anything food, the system is like a web—it's hard to find your way to "safe" ground. And even when you think you are headed in the right direction, you find out that your Better for You Alternative is owned by a company that makes some serious junk, often making you question the better brand you are buying. So, in a way, you may feel like you are damned if you do and damned if you don't. A very legitimate feeling. Who Owns Organic (on following page), compliments of Dr. Phil Howard of Michigan State University, gives you a visual of the web and how Big Food commingles with the more "natural" and organic marketplace.

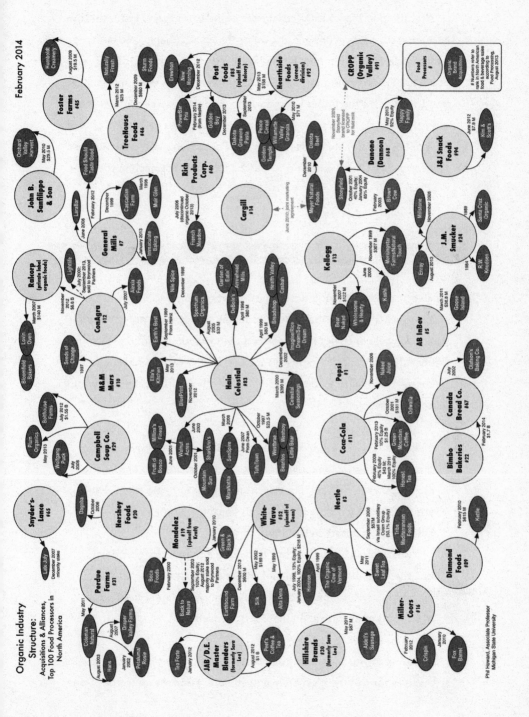

Organic Industry Structure: Acquisitions & Alliances, Top 100 Food Processors in North America

February 2014

Phil Howard, Associate Professor
Michigan State University

According to Mark Kastel, cofounder of the Cornucopia Institute—the NGO that supports economic justice for the local, organic, and authentic family-scale farming community—"food industry acquisitions, big and small, are like a moving target."[1] If you are hungry for more information on "The Who's Who in Big Food and the Good Guys They 'Ate,'" check out Appendix A. If you want to learn more about the real ins and outs of the politics of food, Marion Nestle's *Food Politics*[2] and Wenonah Hauter's *Foodopoly*[3] will surely educate you and churn your stomach at the same time.

Expiration Dating

Believe it or not, there is no federal law requiring expiration dates on anything edible (other than infant formula). So let me clarify the terms that drive your consumption. According to the Natural Resources Defense Council (NRDC), another of my go-to food and environment watchdogs, there are two main categories of labeling—those for the industry and those for consumers:

> "Sell by" dates are a tool for stock control, suggesting when the grocery store should no longer sell products in order to ensure the products still have shelf life after consumers purchase them. They are not meant to communicate with consumers, nor do they indicate the food is bad on that date.
>
> "Best before" and "use by" dates are intended for consumers, but they are often just a manufacturer's estimate of a date after which food will no longer be at peak quality, not an accurate date of spoiling or an indication that food is unsafe.[4]

So how can you realistically use these dates? They say nothing about safety, and for quality, it's merely an estimate. Food waste warrior Dana

Gunders, scientist, avid blogger for the NRDC, and coauthor of *The Dating Game: How Confusing Food Date Labels Lead to Food Waste in America* (in partnership with the Harvard Food Law and Policy Clinic) points out, "The U.S. food dating system is not a system at all. It's a mess. And that mess is leading to a whole lot of perfectly good food going to waste. While to most people it seems that there is a rational, objective system behind the dates we see on our food, it's really more like the Wild West."[5]

The bottom line is that without federal regulations for food dating, you have no way of knowing how these dates have been defined or calculated. Currently, if there is a standard, it is set by state laws (which vary dramatically) or food manufacturers themselves. Once again, food regulations flying by the seat of their pants.

While the NRDC is busy trying to push for change (check out fixfooddates.com), you still need to know how to peruse your pantry and store your food effectively. So follow the basic guidelines set forth in the section titled "What the Fork Is Going On" (page 156) and rely on sight, smell, taste, and basic logic when judging "outdated" food. As Americans waste roughly 40 percent of the food supply per year, I urge you to be part of the solution rather than the problem. For more specifics on safely and unwastefully storing food, check out Appendix C, "Keeping It Fresh, Warding Off Waste."

Now it's time to trash the fat-free salad dressing that your friend insisted you buy but that you hate. And the sugar-free iced tea mix that you picked up for your sister who came to town four weeks ago. How about the soda you buy for special occasions like football night or family gatherings? Or the brightly colored sugared cereals that the kids pester you for? These are the more obvious Grim Reapers, and you want them out (unless they are a Can't Live Without; more on this in sidebar of same name, page 176).

Then dig a little deeper with the section titled "What the Fork Is Going On" as your guide—it's a way to put all your edibles on the witness stand for a further examination so you know what to toss, keep, or replace with Better for You Alternatives. The guide is a checklist, as well as a list of directives, that will counsel you through change. It will help you sort the Grim Reapers from the Keepers. And don't forget to use the Top-Rated Terminator Very Quick Reference Guide (page 149) as needed.

What the Fork Is Going On

THE PANTRY

Dried Herbs and Spices

❑ What's the date? If it's more than two to three years old, toss it (especially if opened).

❑ If there is no expiration date, ask yourself how long you have had it; if it's been hanging around for two to three years, toss it.

❑ Where do you store your herbs and spices? On top of the hot stove? On top of the oven or adjacent to it? If so, then most likely they have lost their flavor (and nutrition) prematurely. My advice, toss them if they are more than a year old. If not, keep them and find them a new home in your kitchen in a cool, dark place.

❑ Does your herb or spice say "non-irradiated"? If not, then presume it is; in an effort not to waste, finish off what you have, then consider non-irradiated for future purchases.

❑ Do you buy reduced-price ground spices and herbs in bulk? If so, watch out for the food fraud factor as described in the sidebar on page 145. In order to aim not to waste, finish them off and buy better next time.

❑ Are herb and spice mixtures and seasoning blends your thing? Often they have a long list of ingredients, many of which aren't even herbs or spices, so investigate ingredients, as TRTs may be lurking. If you don't like what you see, toss.

Oils

- ❑ Where do you keep your oils? Above the hot stove or oven or adjacent to it? If so, they are most likely rancid—oils break down if exposed to too much heat (and light). So take a whiff inside; if the odor is like paint thinner, then toss because it's turned. If there's no odor, then you can most likely salvage it by placing it in the fridge (for olive oil, find a cool, dark place for it).

- ❑ For the oils that remained "safely" in the pantry (away from the heat), if they've been around a while, they very well may be rancid. So take a sniff and if they *do not* stink, move them to your fridge (again, leaving the olive oil out). If they have a stench, even slight, then toss them.

- ❑ Basically all oils, once opened, should be stored in fridge (other than olive oil).

- ❑ Do you buy "light" olive oil because you think it actually has fewer calories? Think again. It's light because it's highly refined, void of flavor, and stripped of valuable nutrition; in order not to waste it, finish what you have, then go for the darker version (versus the "light") next time around.

- ❑ Do you have canola oil, corn oil, or any vegetable oil mix that contains either? Consider them chock-full of GMOs unless they are organic, and happily toss them or aim to finish them and do differently next time around.

- ❑ Do you like almond or walnut oil? FYI, they have a very short shelf life (about three months in the fridge once opened), so if you have used the oil and it's not in a cool area, then most likely it's gone south.

- ❑ What about those big jugs of oils on sale—do you buy? Does it say "100 percent pure olive oil"? If not, chances are it's adulterated. How about those blended bargains? Take a look at what's in your mixture, because it could very well be genetically modified. I say finish what you have unless it is rancid and do better next time.

❏ Do you dive in for that aerosol of oil? Well, most likely it's not just oil in a can but some combination of grease, flavoring, and propellants. Oil straight up does the job just fine; just spread it around with a cloth or brush. Or if you like the spray factor, you can buy one of those pump oil sprayers.

Vinegars

❏ How long have your vinegars been sitting around? Yes, they age like wine and technically have an indefinite shelf life, but once opened, they can turn—your acid will have a sediment, haze, and/or altered color. If so, then most likely its taste has been tampered with. If it is "off," then toss it.

❏ Where do you store your vinegars? If the cap's not twisted tight and it's been sitting near heat and/or light a while (versus in a cool, dark place), then there's a good chance it's bad. Give it a taste and you will know, as it will be extra sour—time to toss.

Condiments and Sauces

❏ Does your ketchup have corn syrup or straight-up sugar? As some form of sugar is inherent in this bottle of red, aim for real sugar versus "corn sugar" (again most likely genetically modified).

❏ Is your mustard colored with yellow dye? How about your pickles or relish? Dyes (and other TRTs) live among many of these condiments. Anything with dye is an easy toss for me.

❏ Is there MSG in any of your bottled sauces, whether salad dressings, teriyaki, or barbecue? What about chemical preservatives (specifically sulfites)? Where is sugar on the ingredient list and what kind is being used? Also, be wary of those artificial colors and flavors. It's some scary stuff, but you decide their destiny.

❏ That dip, soup, or gravy mix most likely contains MSG, lots of artificials, and a multitude of genetically modified ingredients. It's an easy toss in the trash for me.

❑ Is there anything that boasts "sugar-free" or "no sugar added"? What about "fat-free"? Remember, *sugar-free* means it's filled with the fake stuff, and *fat-free* typically means that the fat was replaced with sugar. So, what's this foodstuff's fate?

Canned Goods (Bottles and Boxes, Too)

❑ Do you have canned veggies, even bottled ones? Most likely sugar is added to the mix in some form, and even chemical preservatives. And don't forget the infamous canned corn that is most likely genetically modified. Keep and finish, deciding to do better next time, or pass along to the food pantry.

❑ Tomatoes in a can or jar are typically okay, just look out for the added sugar in many brands; for sure finish what you have and do better next time.

❑ Do you do broths, soups, or brews (like chili and/or other bean dishes slammed into a can)? Watch out for MSG, anything artificial, and GMO ingredients like soy (as in soy protein isolates or textured vegetable protein). If the product has any kind of meat, wonder where it came from. You determine its destiny.

❑ Speaking of meat in a can, whether straight up or wrapped in ravioli, surely consider where the ground round came from and all the other stuff mixed in to make the blend. Again, what's its destiny?

❑ Many canned beans come straight up, but there are plenty with chemical preservatives like EDTA—not too offensive but totally unnecessary. So finish what you have and buy better next time.

❑ Canned or jarred fruits are typically loaded with some form of sugar—most typically the GMO corn syrup variety. You determine its destiny.

❑ If you love jam, is your fruit preserve pounded with added sugar? Fruit is sweet without being supplemented with sugar (though a tad is just fine). So finish it and buy better next time. If it's sugar-free, it's surely packed with superficial sweetness. This is an easy toss in the trash.

❑ How about maple syrup? Is your maple the real deal or corn syrup artificially flavored with maple goodness? Definitely deliver to the "dump" if fake.

❑ When you buy nut butter, whether peanut, almond, or soy, is it simply nuts ground with a little salt or is the "butter" loaded with sugar and/or hydrogenated oils? You may find oil added to your nut butter (and not the hydrogenated version)—is it canola or cottonseed? If so, it is most likely the GMO variety unless organic. Figure out how you want to navigate nut butters.

❑ Anything canned, bottled, or boxed, once opened, can last days to weeks. Use sight, smell, and taste here.

Pasta, Grains, and Dried Beans

❑ Whether pasta is wheat (white or whole) or a gluten-free option, buy what you like; just beware of corn pastas, as many use the GMO variety.

❑ Do you like quick rice or quick any other grain? Note that they are "fast" because they are partially cooked or masticated and potentially void of valuable nutrition. You can pass them to the food pantry if unopened.

❑ You can't go wrong with whole grains or beans in a bag, so definitely keep these (unless they are discolored and have been hanging around for more than three years).

❑ Do you buy bleached flours? Or those with added nutrients or preservatives? Scrutinize your labels here and decide which way you want to go.

❑ How long have your flours been around? Do you keep them airtight in a cool dry place once opened? If not and they've been hanging around for more than a year, they are most likely losers. If they have been recently opened, keep them in the fridge or freezer for freshness (bleached flours and flour mixes may last longer and do fine in a cool, dark place).

Breads and Bakery

❑ Where do you keep your bread products—in a designated drawer or the refrigerator? Typically breads stale faster when kept in the fridge (especially those that are fresh baked) but at the same time, if void of chemical preservatives, breads do tend to spoil more quickly in the long run. Aim to keep them at room temperature for a few days once opened then toss in the fridge to maintain freshness. A quick pop in the toaster oven will have it back to tender in no time.

❑ Do you opt for the common white or whole wheat? Either way, both can be loaded with TRTs, including more sugar than needed, chemical preservatives, and GMO ingredients.

❑ Does your bread product or baked good boast "whole grain" goodness? It may not be whole grain (meaning that the edible parts—the bran, germ, and endosperm remain) unless it bears the sticker from the Whole Grains Council (see chapter 11). While processed foods made with whole grains are your better choice, intact grains (like oats and rice) are truly the best option. But for bread and baked goods, aim for foods with the Whole Grains emblem (if you can find them); however, don't convince yourself that a sugary muffin made with wholeness is supercharged for health support.

❑ Do you have any bread gone stale? If so, cut it up to make some croutons or toss it in the freezer for crunch at a later date so as not to waste it.

❑ What about those boxes of bread crumbs, croutons, or simple stuffing? Typically the TRTs abound, so buyer beware. Toss or pass to the food pantry.

❑ And when you buy baked goods, whether scones, muffins, coffee cake, or doughnuts, vet through the ingredients, as TRTs are all too common—and don't think that you are buying anything other than a sweet treat. You determine its destiny.

Cereals

❑ Do you have the colored sugary cereals for yourself or your little loved ones? You should know by now that most cereal offers little to no real nutrition (despite all the claims), so think twice about sucking down all that sugar, the risky rainbow, and other TRTs each morning.

❑ Watch out for the boxes that brag too much, because they are most likely phonies. You may get some fiber or "added-value" protein from cereal, but what does that come with? Sugar and other TRTs. You determine the destiny of your crunch.

❑ Any cereal that boasts high protein is commonly laced with soy, and often the GMO variety; get your protein from beans, nuts, seeds, or animal foods, not cereal.

❑ Steer clear of small packets of hot cereal, as most are loaded with sugar, artificial flavors, and even artificial colors; you can pass these to the food pantry.

❑ If anything boasts "sugar-free," be on the lookout for artificial sweetness.

❑ Just because it's granola doesn't mean that it is super healthy. Most commercial granolas are loaded with sugar and calories. Do you have a bag? If so, check out the sugar content—if it has more than 5 grams per serving, rethink your granola.

❑ If you have that bag of whole-grain cereal goodness like steel-cut oats, rolled oats, or muesli, I applaud you. Keep and eat.

Nuts and Seeds

❑ If you have nuts and seeds raw or roasted with or without salt, then you are good. Just check their freshness, as once opened, they should ideally live in your fridge to stay super fresh.

❑ Watch out for the mixes with added oil like cottonseed or canola— these are most likely genetically modified; finish what you have and do better next time.

❑ Flavored nuts are often loaded with sugar, MSG, and other TRTs, so my thought is to toss these or pass them to the food pantry if they are unopened.

❑ Do you buy trail mix with sugared fruit or colored chocolate thinking that it's healthy because it's a "trail mix"? Think again. The same nutty stuff from earlier applies, but you are now dealing with unnecessary sugar (from the fruit and the candy), perhaps even sulfite preservatives in the dried goodness, and of course dyes if the mix have sightings of red, yellow, or blue. I would trash these.

Snacks

❑ Does your crunch—chips, pretzels, or crackers—come with trans fats? More often than not it's some form of canola, cottonseed, or corn oil, and typically of the GMO variety. Even if not hydrogenated, it is mostly likely from the same GMO source. Take note of any other TRTs too. Reaper or keeper?

❑ If your crunch is flavored, as in sour cream and onion potato chips, watch out for added sugar, artificial flavors and colors, and chemical preservatives—all very common. Consider these an easy toss.

❑ Sweets like cookies have all the same stuff as the crunch but with a lot more sugar. And don't think a packaged cookie can boast good nutrition (though not all are created equal); I suspect that this may be an easy toss.

❑ Many granola bars boast better nutrition but are just as bad as cookies high in sugar, fat, and other TRTs, so watch out for the health claims, as they will surely persuade you to think otherwise; it's totally your call here.

❑ And, of course, if any of the sweet stuff brags of being "sugar-free," it's most likely filled with the artificials. This is an easy toss for me.

❑ Make sure your dried fruit leaves the added sugar behind—most of them don't. And be on the lookout for those dried bursts of flavor (like apricots) with chemical preservatives, namely sulfites.

❑ And what about those fruity snacks? Do you buy them because your little loved one begs? Well, most of them aren't related to any fruit; they are more like glorified candy—and typically they are chock-full of TRTs. Terrible for teeth and totally tossable.

Baking

❑ Watch out for many of those mainstream mixes, as they are loaded with artificial everything; I beg you to toss them, as I will introduce you to much better options.

❑ Many chocolate chips, or any chips for that matter, are artificially flavored; finish what you have if you must.

❑ Whether sprinkles, frosting, decorative icings, or food dye, consider this a significant rainbow of risk. Also note the artificial flavors and choice GMO ingredients in these colorful combos. I beg you to bash them in the trash.

❑ Watch out for the extracts. Do you have pure vanilla extract or vanilla-flavored extract? They are very different. Go for the pure. The same holds true for all other extracts.

❑ Do you have those all-purpose baking mixes? Investigate the ingredient list, as trans fats could be listed (among a few other curious choices). If yuck, then toss them. If not, keep them in the fridge if they are opened.

❑ Make sure your sugar reads "pure cane sugar," otherwise its source could be GMO sugar beets.

Beverages

❑ Do you have any beverage powders? If so, most likely they are some combination of sugar and artificial flavors, colors, and even sweeteners (real or fake). It's time to say good-bye.

❑ Juice is sugar water, so drink wisely. If it says "sugar-free," buyer beware as it's absolutely artificial. It may have some fake flavors and colors too. Also, note that sugar can very well come from GMO sugar beets. This is a no-brainer—bye-bye.

❑ Do you stock soda straight up or diet? How about sugary sports drinks? Watch out for the corn syrup and fake colors, flavors, and of course sweeteners. These are totally tossable.

❑ Do you like alternative milks like soy? Unless it's organic, it is most likely from GMO soy. Also, keep an eye out for added sugar in all alternative milks, even rice, almond, hemp, coconut, and so on.

❑ Do you dabble in protein powders or any kind of "muscle-making milk"? Most are loaded with sugar (artificial too), fake flavors, and more. So consumer, be cautious. I advise taking it to the trash.

Candy

❑ Do you keep candy in the house? If so, you know it's loaded with sugar (or perhaps one of the artificials). But what about all of the other TRTs, namely the fake flavors and colors? It's up to you.

Are you overwhelmed? If not, consider yourself unique. The process of any makeover can be mind-twisting and quite emotional. But a huge congrats to you, as you made it through the pantry—probably the hardest part. Right now, your food should be sorted into two piles, Grim Reapers and Keepers, and perhaps along the way, you became so disgusted that you just tossed tons in the trash. All good. Take a deep breath; next up are the fridge and freezer.

If you are exhausted from the pantry part, that is understandable and totally fine. Leave the fridge and freezer for another day. Trust me, it's not going to run away. But you may if you don't take a breather. If you opt for the much-needed break, jump to chapter 13 before you close up shop for the day.

If you want to forge ahead then the next step is going through the icebox and identifying the Grim Reapers and the Keepers. It's no different from what you did with the pantry, except you may want to sort through while the food still hangs out in the frostiness.

The Fridge and Freezer

The day after the infamous Hurricane Sandy hit my East Coast hometown, I sadly removed everything from my powerless refrigerator and freezer. Cooler in hand to keep what I could, I readily tossed what was no longer trustworthy, and in the process, I came across that jar of relish that was opened six months earlier and had a stench; the barely used yet incredibly unsavory bottle of salad dressing that my husband bought when I was out of town; the flat seltzer; and the freezer-burned "better for you" waffles that my son Hunter begged for when we went food shopping but were eaten once. Funny, I thought my cooler was squeaky clean.

Even without Sandy, it is time for you to do the same. Ditch the old, the tired, and the yuck. Make room for the yum. And pick up some simple storage tips along the way to keep your food as cool and fresh as can be to limit waste (and reduce your food bill).

What the Fork Is Going On

FRIDGE

Produce (Fruits, Vegetables, and Herbs)

❑ Where is your produce from? Somewhere overseas or the United States of America? Maybe even local? A little advice: try to eat foods that are in season and grown as close to home as possible. They will have more nutrition for sure. Keep what you have and do better next time.

❑ Do you buy conventional produce? If so, are any of your selections on the Environmental Working Group's Dirty Dozen Plus™ (a list of the produce that retains the highest level of pesticide residue, available at ewg.org or as a smartphone app)? If you consume tons of items on that list, aim to buy organic next time around if possible.

❑ Where do you keep your produce? In your crisper drawers on the bottom or just tossed anywhere in your fridge? If anywhere, what was once fresh is most likely dying a fast death, so take a look and see what you can salvage.

❑ Is your produce molded? Are your carrots limp, and your greens and herbs wilted, slimy, or browned? If so, it's time to toss them. But wait, limp and wilted are still okay and can be used to make a soup of sorts (check out chapter 18 for a recipe or two).

❑ Is your fruit bruised or a little sketchy? Most people will toss imperfection, but I urge you to keep it, cut it up, and use it for a smoothie (see the recipes in chapter 18). Always know that you can freeze berries, bananas, grapes, kiwi, papaya, pineapple, mango, melon, and watermelon as they make great snacks and are delish in a blended beverage.

❑ Best bet is to keep what's truly alive living, store fruits in a low-humidity crisper drawer (most fridges these days have one); vegetables are best in the high-humidity drawer. As greens and herbs are super delicate, I urge you to wrap them in a wet paper towel and put them in an airtight bag or container. Check out NRDC's Refrigerator Demystified (page 174) to develop a better relationship with your coolbox.

Deli and Meats

❑ What's really in your deli drawer? If you purchased deli meats at any old grocer, most likely they are loaded with nitrates and nitrites, fillers, and who knows what else. And are you into the fake meats, as in vegetarian or vegan "meat" options? Highly processed soy and chemical flavors can be just as bad. It's up to you to decide what to do.

❑ The previous note holds true for the plain old hot dog too. Hmm, do you really know where that "meat" comes from? Better options exist, even for the hot dog. You decide. . . .

❑ Bacon is notorious for being full of added nitrates and nitrites, so beware. And if you have a half-opened package, did you safely store it in an airtight plastic bag? If not, it could very well be some shade of gray, and it's rubbish.

- ❑ Speaking of meat, did you check the date on that chicken you bought for dinner a few days ago but never cooked? How about the ground beef that you bought six months ago but just defrosted. Many times meat goes bad before the date or if it is stored for too long in the fridge—and you know by smell and color. By the way, your meat should *never* have a stench or be slightly gray or discolored. If either of these applies, consider it a goner.

- ❑ Do you know anything about the origin of your meats? Were the animals humanely raised? Were hormones and antibiotics used? Finish what you have and do better next time using the "Decoding Food Marketing Madness: The Funny (and Not-So-Funny) Label Lingo" in chapter 11 as a guide.

- ❑ Do you fancy fish? Is it from the United States? Is it wild or farmed, and if it is from a fishery, do you know anything about the aquaculture environment or how your finny friends were cared for? Your guess is as good as mine. How long has it been sitting around? Even if you just bought it, there should be *no* smell whatsoever. If so, it's turned, so go ahead and toss it.

Dairy (Milk, Butter, Cheese, Yogurt, Other) and Eggs

- ❑ Who's making your milk or milk products? Has it hailed from cows that were humanely treated and drug-free? What about your egg-laying hens? Were they truly pasture raised? Most likely the answer is no, and you know it because the package doesn't allude to anything about animals, or if it does, you have little idea what it really means. You can refer to chapter 11 for some guidance.

- ❑ Your buttery spread should just be cream and perhaps some salt. But many brands today add "natural" flavors and colors such as annatto ("natural" but concerning for some) to keep it looking buttery. Finish feasting and try for better the next time around.

❑ Cream cheese really should just be a modest combination of milk, cream, salt, and perhaps plant-based fillers/stabilizers like guar or locust bean gum. Does your cream cheese have just that, or is it complemented by flavor, whether natural or artificial, plus chemical preservatives? If so, you decide.

❑ Do you do margarine? Chances are it's laced with trans fats and plenty of other TRTs. This is a no-brainer—bash in the trash. Trans fat–free spreads are most likely loaded with other not-so-loving loot, so scrutinize.

❑ Do you have crusty cheese in your deli drawer? Or a chunk that was nibbled at but improperly stored so it's got some green growing? Cheese needs to be tightly wrapped. Toss it if it's turned.

❑ And what's in your cheese? Is it real cheese or processed "cheese food"? Many cheeses, whether slices (to some extent), shreds, dips, or sprays, can have added flavor, typically "natural"; color like annatto (again, "natural" but concerning for some); chemical preservatives (like sulfites); mold inhibitors like natamycin (which can come from a GMO bacteria source); and anticaking agents like cornstarch (most likely from GMO corn). It's good to know what's inside so you can decide if you want to ditch what's absolutely unnecessary.

❑ Whether your yogurt is organic or not, are you buying the package of promise that is sugar-free or has a zillion probiotics to purge your gut? Are you dazzled by the fabulous flavors? Something to ponder—yogurt is essentially fermented milk, and with fermentation comes healthy bacteria (as in probiotics), but the sugar added to most yogurts today can render those healthy bacteria ineffective. Yup, sugar can promote the growth of unhealthy bacteria, so if you buy the sugared yogurts, you could be zeroed out. Also, watch out for the sugar substitutes, chemical flavors, and even color. Best bet, be on guard and do better next time.

❑ Both sour cream and cottage cheese, unless flavored with fakeness, are typically inoffensive.

❑ And do you buy into the eggs with oodles of omega fats? Your hens are being fed flax to give them that "healthy" fatty boost. But know this: You are probably paying considerably more for these ovals for a benefit that you could get from food like walnuts. Enough with the fortified foods; just fetch the necessary fat straight from nuts, flax, fish, or fish oil or truly pasture-raised animal foods that are naturally higher in the omegas.

❑ If your eggs have been sitting around for a while, do a freshness test by plopping them in a bowl of water. If they sink but stand upright, then boil them (they are about to go bad). If unfit for consumption, they will float to the top.

Prepared Foods/Leftovers

❑ Are you a purchaser of prepared foods, and if so, are they still fresh? Take a whiff, even a taste if you can't tell (you won't keel over). If your food was truly fresh when you bought it, it should keep for an average of three days. If not, it might not have been that perky when you bought it—a big bummer. Make sure your choices are super fresh when you purchase (if you are in the prepared-foods section of a store, ask for a taste of what you intend to buy to check for freshness).

❑ Are you a leftover lover? If so, check out your inventory with some sniffing and tiny tasting. If it's rotten, toss it. Keep leftovers in the fridge for an average of three days. After that, move them to the freezer for up to three months. In other words, save what you can now.

Beverages

❑ Is your fridge adorned with opened bottles of brightly colored drinks or soda? Need I say more?

❑ Are your bevvies, like juice (even if boasting great nutrition), teas, lemonade, limeade, or flavored and sweetened milks, stacked with sugar? Have some good old water or some juice cut with water instead.

❑ Do you drink "functional" beverages boasting no end to nutritional benefits? These can take the form of sports drinks, teas and tonics, coconut water, aloe vera drinks, chia coolers, and even kombucha. Some can have unnecessary added sugar; flavors, whether "natural" or artificial; and even chemical preservatives, especially with aloe vera. So buyer beware.

❑ Do you like tasteful seltzer? A word to the wise: Those seltzers are razzed with "natural" flavors. How about plain seltzer with a squeeze of lemon or lime?

FREEZER

Produce (Fruits and Vegetables)

❑ Contrary to popular belief, frozen produce can be a good thing. Fruits and veggies are picked at peak freshness and frozen with the nutrition in. So keep a variety around, but make sure that they don't have freezer burn.

❑ Do you buy the kind of frozen fruit with added sugar? Buyer beware.

❑ Most frozen potatoes, whether fries or tots, are enhanced with chemical preservatives, flavors of some sort, and possible GMO ingredients. Please do better next time.

Meat, Poultry, and Fish

❑ Think about where your animal foods came from and what's really in them (see chapter 11, "Decoding Marketing Madness: The Funny (and Not-So-Funny) Label Lingo") and determine their destiny.

❑ How long have your meats been in the freezer? If meat is really dark and gray, to the trash it should go. If you see bright white on poultry, think freezer burn and toss.

❑ How long has your fish been there? Is it bright white (usually indicating freezer burn) and does it have a funky odor? To reiterate: Much of the fish you buy "fresh" at the market was frozen and thawed for sale to you. So it's best not put it back in the freezer when you get home, as fish that has been frozen twice (or maybe even more) doesn't fly in the culinary or nutrition department.

Prepared Foods/Leftovers

❑ Are you a frozen-dinner fanatic? If so, dig into the ingredients, as most are loaded with the TRTs plus tons of sodium. There are better options to buy for sure.

❑ And how long have you had these meals and sides around? Perhaps a year or two? If so, then toss. Best to let them hang around for less than a year.

❑ Do you go for the weight-loss meal selections? They may boast fewer calories, but often their ingredient list is incredibly offensive, containing many TRTs. You decide. . . .

❑ What about veggie burgers? Do you buy into the rubbery round? Just because it's veggie does not mean that it's healthy, even if it's organic. There are lots of GMO ingredients (in the nonorganic sort), fillers, and chemical flavors in most beefless burgers. Your choice.

❑ Check your leftovers for freezer burn. You'd be surprised at how quickly this once-fresh delish can take a nosedive. If it's fuzzy with frost, then toss it.

Breads and Bakery

❑ Are you the sort to buy half-baked bread, then plop it in the oven like it's your own? Scrutinize the ingredients here, as many of these loaves contain multiple TRTs.

❑ Do you have those burger buns stashed away from the summer before with freezer burn? They may not look gross but they surely taste it, so into the trash they should go.

❑ What about baked goods, including waffles, muffins, doughnuts, and more? Are you buying into the BS on the box? What about the TRTs? Breakfast items like this don't carry real nutrition, so your best bet is to avoid the brainwash.

Sweet Treats

❑ Does your ice cream (dairy or nondairy) have freezer burn? And where do the TRTs live in this creamy wonder?

❑ Are you one for those "skinny" desserts? Well, talk about junk—you are better off with a small bowl of real-deal ice cream, as most likely, many TRTs live in these chemical creatures.

❑ On the ice pop front, watch out for those fake flavors and colors, and don't fall prey to the "sugar-free" solution. This is just more chemical cuisine. So, what will it be?

❑ And if you opt for frozen cookie dough, watch out for those TRTs because there can be plenty of them.

Now that you have screened the items in your igloo, put your Grim Reapers on the table with those from the pantry, embrace the Keepers, and take this opportunity to wipe that cool box clean (be sure not to leave perishables uncool for too long). As you will inevitably reorganize, I encourage you to use the Refrigerator Demystified guide on the next page, compliments of the Natural Resources Defense Council,[6] to learn how to store food safely and effectively limit waste. In the end, limiting waste adds wampum to your wallet. Now what to do? Rehab Strategies to the rescue . . .

THE REFRIGERATOR
Demystified

Up to 40 percent of food in the U.S. is never eaten. Stocking your fridge with these tips will help make a dent in food waste, saving you money while you do it.

NRDC
The Earth's Best Defense

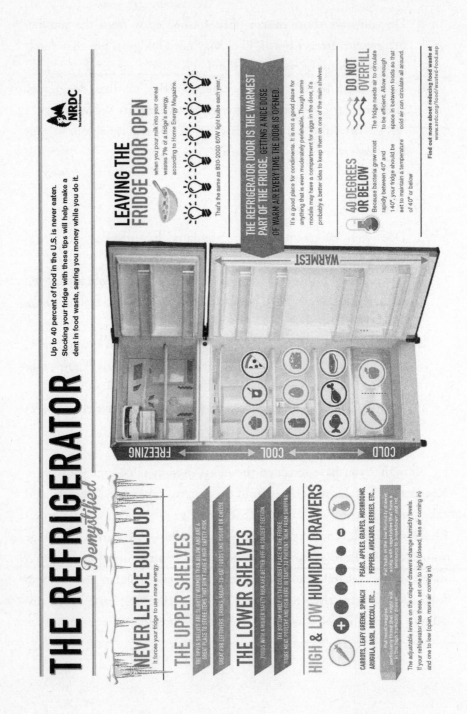

NEVER LET ICE BUILD UP
It forces your fridge to use more energy.

THE UPPER SHELVES
THE UPPER SHELVES ARE SLIGHTLY WARMER THAN BELOW AND ARE A GREAT PLACE TO STORE ITEMS THAT DON'T HAVE A HIGH SAFETY RISK

GREAT FOR LEFTOVERS, DRINKS, READY-TO-EAT FOODS LIKE YOGURT OR CHEESE

THE LOWER SHELVES
FOODS WITH A HIGHER SAFETY RISK ARE BETTER OFF IN COLDEST SECTION

THE BOTTOM SHELF IS THE COLDEST PLACE IN THE FRIDGE. STORE MEAT, POULTRY AND FISH HERE IN TRAYS TO PREVENT THEM FROM DRIPPING.

HIGH & LOW HUMIDITY DRAWERS

Put fruits in the low humidity drawer, along with vegetables that have a tendency to breakdown and rot.

CARROTS, LEAFY GREENS, SPINACH, ARUGULA, BASIL, BROCCOLI, ETC...

PEARS, APPLES, GRAPES, MUSHROOMS, PEPPERS, AVOCADOS, BERRIES, ETC...

Put leafy vegetables and those that might wilt in the high humidity drawer.

The adjustable levers on the crisper drawers change humidity levels.

If your refrigerator has these, set one to high (closed, less air coming in) and one to low (open, more air coming in).

FREEZING · **COOL** · **COLD**

WARMEST

LEAVING THE FRIDGE DOOR OPEN

when you pour your milk into your cereal wastes 7% of a fridge's energy, according to Home Energy Magazine."

That's the same as 830-2000 60W light bulbs each year.

THE REFRIGERATOR DOOR IS THE WARMEST PART OF THE FRIDGE. GETTING A NICE DOSE OF WARM AIR EVERY TIME THE DOOR IS OPENED.

It's a good place for condiments. It is not a good place for anything that is even moderately perishable. Though some models may have a compartment for eggs in the door, it's probably a better idea to keep them on one of the main shelves.

40 DEGREES OR BELOW
Because bacteria grow most rapidly between 40° and 140°, your fridge should be set to maintain a temperature of 40° or below

DO NOT OVERFILL
The fridge needs air to circulate to be efficient. Allow enough space in between foods so that cold air can circulate all around.

Find out more about reducing food waste at www.nrdc.org/food/wasted-food.asp

CHAPTER 13

Rehab Strategies: Out with the Bad, In with the Better

Whenever I'm visiting someone near and dear, I often hear, "Just do me a favor and don't look in my pantry."

It's enough that I am inside the pantries, fridges, and freezers of my clients, so when it comes to family and friends, my rule of thumb is to *try* to keep my mouth shut. And most of the time I succeed.

But sometimes I don't. One summer, a dear high school friend whom I hadn't seen in years was proudly showing me around his new home, kitchen first, and I slipped (and I don't mean ass on the floor).

"Hey, Stef, check out my awesome pantry!" Well, he opened up this sizable closet and I gasped. Literally. I just couldn't help myself. He is a cancer survivor and has four kids.

I took one look at him, with my jaw dropped and eyes bulging, and said (in a slightly elevated tone), "What are you thinking?"

He immediately closed the pantry closet and told me to zip it. He said his wife did all the shopping and if I said anything, I would be kicked out of the house. So I zipped it but did say this: "For every bit of garbage you have in your pantry, and you have quite a bit, there is a healthier alternative." He yessed me, I kept my mouth closed, and we vacationed at his home for three days. But to this day, our conversation still continues.

My point is that anything and everything food is a charged topic. And right now, you may be feeling edgy. Perhaps motivated but with a little pit in your stomach? Or once motivated but now slightly pissed off? I get it because I work with people like you every day. So please trust me when I say that shifting your edible choices and habits is by no measure a death sentence, but rather a life sentence, and you can still enjoy the foods you love— just please allow me to introduce you to the Better for You Alternatives. I promise you that for every bit of unhealthy, there is a better option that tastes equally good, or maybe even better. And if it doesn't taste as good, you have one of two choices: Suck it up, knowing that your palate will adjust, and embrace the fact that you are eating something that is more health supportive; or make the junk food a Can't Live Without exception. It is really up to you.

Can't Live Without

As a kid, I spent many winter weekends in Vermont skiing with my family. It was on these trips that a family tradition was born—before my brother and I headed for the slopes, my mom stuffed our jacket pockets with Haribo gummy bears. These delicious bursts of chewy flavor were filled with sugar and food dye, but I loved them then and still do now, and nothing is going to get in the way of our "relationship." Lucky for me, I have found a much healthier alternative in Yummy Earth gummy bears, but nothing can replace the taste of my childhood.

You all have those Can't Live Withouts, whether founded on traditions or simply "I like the taste of a *really bad for me* food" like a Big Mac. Either way, it is okay and quite healthy to have foods that you just can't live without—life is about balance. If at all possible, try to go for the Better for You Alternatives (like Yummy Earth gummies). Making compromises with the foods you choose is a tricky task, whether for yourself or your loved ones.

Know this—extremes do no one any good. Many years ago I had a client who was utterly frustrated because her eight-year-old daughter was exposed to and devoured junk food (hot dogs, pizza, cookies, cakes, candy, and soda) at birthday parties. My first question was, "Do you ever give her these foods, even their healthier versions, at home?"

Her reply was, "Absolutely not!" Dear readers, we live in a world where you can't keep little ones (or yourselves) sheltered from junk food. If you restrict too much, kids will rebel (and so will you). So dabble in "forbidden food" without the guilt.

So do I practice what I preach? Absolutely! And I imagine that many of you want to know how I do it, so here it is: Ninety percent of the time, I consume foods void of the TRTs whether at home or otherwise. I leave the 10 percent for the occasional product that might have a GMO ingredient in it (hard to avoid), those eggs that I have to grab at the local supermarket that I know came from hens that were not humanely raised or for meals out (plus that Haribo gummy bear—hey, I'm human). So generally speaking, we eat everything from kale to candy, but most of our food is made with the purest ingredients (yes, this can be done).

When we are outside the home, I have learned to loosen the reins a bit. Birthday parties are a free-for-all. At this stage, my kids are making conscious choices for themselves. For school, I have no worries—healthy food is central to their place of education. As for summer camp, it can be a bit of an unsavory food fest, but I work with the camp director on what my boys can eat (the chicken-like nuggets are *not* okay, nor are the incandescent ice pops) and help them navigate the choices themselves. When we go to the movies, all bets are off, and the kids go to the local candy store to get a small bag of whatever they want. What it boils down to is making educated choices—don't let ignorance be bliss when it comes to your food consumption. Moderation is truly my mantra (I have done all the extremes and am over it).

So now look at your Grim Reapers and decide what items you and yours *really* can't live without. Is it that diet soda that you drink once a day or the package of artificial sweetness that puts a stamp on skinny whether in coffee or tea? What about a Twinkie? I can honestly tell you that I think those are the only foodstuffs that there are no real replacements for. Whether you have a laundry list of Can't Live Without foods, or you *really want* to go for the gold with the makeover, there is a way to navigate.

1. Your ideal strategy is to replace 100 percent of your Can't Live Without foods with Better for You Alternatives (see Appendix B, "Common Food Brands and Recommended Alternatives")— though if diet soda, artificial sweeteners, and Twinkies are on the list, I have no real solution here other than to kiss those puppies good-bye.

2. If you can't achieve #1, try to limit yourself to one to three Can't Live Without foods, whether daily or weekly. You may start out daily and then realize that reducing your intake isn't as bad as you thought (especially knowing what you now know). If you are silly for superficial sweetness, perhaps put one packet rather than two in your coffee each day.

3. Finally, if you just can't let go of *any* of your Can't Live Without foods, how about trying to at least cut your consumption in half? So if you're like my Coke-loving client who sucked down three a day when we first started working together, try two a day for one month, then one a day for the next month, and take it from there. For the other Can't Live Withouts, use the same strategy. Basically you are still eating what you enjoy (despite the potential consequences), but you are greatly reducing your intake.

No matter what your strategy is, you are doing better than you were, and I applaud you for that. Remember, small changes can make big everyday differences.

Okay, so now that your food is sorted, it's time to offer some tactile rehab strategies:

1. Feng Shui Your Food—Clear the crumbs from your cubbies and feel free to give your fridge a good clean. If you are so inclined, remove the shelves and drawers for a fridge "detail." If you're not up for the "superwash," then aim to clear out everything from the sticky syrup and crusty milk to particles of produce. Then put the Keepers back where they belong. If you are an organization fanatic like me, feel free to pull out that label maker for some food signage—it can offer a little consumption clarity (though I do it only for my pantry).

2. Reaper Rescue Guide—At this point, your Grim Reapers alone should be staring you in the face. Using the guide above, write down every product (including brand name, like Jell-O) that contains too many TRTs to bear and determine if you can live without it. Then you can address the third column, the Better for You Alternatives, when your list of items that you'd be willing to replace is complete.

3. Can't Live Without—All I ask is that you make your choices from a place of knowledge rather than ignorance regarding the foods that you *must have* (but you know aren't really doing yourself any good).

4. Your Local Food Pantry—Once your Reaper Rescue Guide is complete, toss what you no longer want or need and pack away the unopened products for your local food pantry.

Now, with list in hand, toss any remaining unwanted and start to scan Appendix B, "Common Food Brands and Recommended Alternatives." This will give you an idea of the Better for You Alternatives that actually exist. And perhaps ease your possible pain just a little.

REAPER RESCUE GUIDE

PRODUCT/BRAND	CAN YOU LIVE WITHOUT?	THE BETTER FOR YOU ALTERNATIVE (SEE APPENDIX B FOR GUIDANCE)
(sample) Jell-O	Yes	Simply Delish Jel Desserts

Getting the Family on Board

Change is not easy. And while *you* may be ready, those you live with may not be. Chapter 16 is devoted to strategies for introducing the Better for You Alternatives, but until then, I would like to offer this as warm-up:

1. For the skeptical spouse or mate, ask them to read *What the Fork*; if they don't want to, share excerpts or simply start gabbing about what you are learning. They may start to snuggle up to the idea of shifting with you.

2. If you have kids, definitely start talking about what you are learning. For instance, if your kid asks for a colorful food product, share a little info on food dyes with them. When you pop into a market with your child, grab some products and start reading ingredient lists with them and turn them on to the Environmental Working Group's Food Database™ (kids love apps and anything electronic).

3. Once you have given your partner and/or kids sufficient warm-up time (perhaps the amount of time it takes you to read this book or even longer), tell them that you are going to do a food makeover because you want everyone to be as healthy as they can be. And you know you can *all* do better.

4. This may be met with, "Don't take my Oreos away" or "I want my Kraft mac and cheese." Reassure them that you are not taking anything away, but replacing those items with healthier options, so chocolate sandwich cookies and mac and cheese are still okay, but you are aiming for more conscious consumption.

5. For partners who put up a fight, they can do as they please, but tell them that you will set aside a cabinet (and cooler shelf) for their Can't Live Withouts. If you have children, say this to your other half: "Please help me foster healthy habits in our children; I now understand how important it is for their overall well-being, and your support is very critical."

6. For the feisty and furious young folk, it is your job as a parent to provide a variety of healthy foods for your children, so I urge you to take a stand. Newsflash: You are the boss—so *you* set the rules. You can say this to the kid who is old enough and has a strong voice: "There will be new food rules. If you absolutely hate the healthier alternatives, then I am happy to negotiate, but you are required to try everything. When you are outside the house, you can do as you please. It is your health, your choice." Over time, this child typically jumps on board.

You are officially ready for Supermarket Strategies. You may feel overwhelmed, and you may be thinking, "OMG, I can't believe I just threw all that food away." Or, "How the heck am I ever going to be able to find replacements for everything?" Maybe it's "I feel like I am in a food minefield with all these labels. How am I going to know how to navigate?" And of course there is the concern that eating more healthfully will cost you more.

Well, allow me to enlighten you:

1. You threw away food that is utterly unhealthy. You now know the ugly truth, so why would you want to continue chomping on crap?

2. You can reference Appendix B, "Common Food Brands and Recommended Alternatives," for the better brands and know that there are alternatives. And when you go to your food bazaar, the better brands will most likely be waiting.

3. Section Three, "Supermarket Strategies," will teach you how to navigate the aisles in your market of munch.

4. Here is a thought about food cost: Any way you slice it, you will pay for what you eat. If you pay up front (meaning at the grocery store), then you have a better chance of being healthy. If you pay on the back end (meaning at the doctor's office), what you eat is most likely costing you much more. So you decide.

Supermarket Strategies

While I love peeking in people's pantries, one of the best parts of helping them make over their munch is when we shop till we drop. I rarely buy clothes, but I do shop for food, whether solo, with my kids, or with a client. It is seriously one of my favorite things to do. Call me crazy.

Many years ago I had the pleasure of working with an accomplished chef and his wife. He is the executive culinarian of five well-known restaurants, and she had a kidney disease. They were on board to do better than they were doing, and *she* had no choice. I work with all sorts, but an accomplished chef—c'mon, what could I *really* teach him about food that he didn't already know?

As is standard with my clients (after the initial evaluation in their home), we visited a local supermarket for a two-hour shopping education tour. In this case, little did I know that the mister was in for quite a shocker. I gabbed about the foods found in his home that had elevated TRT levels, from junky cereals and soda to sauces and condiments, and pointed out the Better for You Alternatives as we perused the aisles. This master chef was flabbergasted, as he thought that many of his choices were pretty healthy, from animal foods to the bottles of culinary flavor. To his credit, since then he has made a significant change not only in family food but also in what he does for each and every eatery he commands.

My point is that even someone so in the know about food was astonished by what he *didn't know* and was quite confused. So I imagine that you will be too. How could you not? Traditional supermarkets carry anywhere from fifteen thousand to sixty thousand products, according to the U.S. Department of the Treasury's Community Development Finance Institution's report "Understanding the Grocery Industry" (2011).[1] Honestly, that alone is enough to spin your head when you march into the market.

And get this: There is also a hidden war of the aisles, whereby food companies compete for the best shelf real estate and pay top dollar for it. So what does that mean for you? Well, figure that the companies with the most money will have the best property explaining why their products will be at eye level—yours and your loved ones'. And sadly, those companies are primarily the ones whose commodities contain the infamous Top-Rated Terminators. You are bound to get sucked in.

To add a little more mess to the mix, roughly fifteen thousand *new food products* are introduced *per year*. Yet more decisions to make. Folks, you are in an uphill battle. And you will continue to fight that battle until *you*, the consumer, start demanding Keepers versus Grim Reapers and insisting on food transparency. In other words, take *What the Fork* to heart and start making a difference with your dollars.

The goal here is very simple—to furnish you with aisle-by-aisle action-ables for sorting through these overwhelming markets (and even the not-so-imposing ones) and to *finally* set the record straight about navigating nourishment. I'll also give some excellent strategies to get your family on board.

Cartoon Characters and Crappy Food

My son Jack has been my supermarket sidekick since birth. Perusing the aisles, we talk about food and read labels, picking and choosing the familiar and sometimes not-so-familiar edibles to buy.

With me as his mom, he has no choice but to be aware of where his food comes from and what's in it. But he is still a kid. And I want him to be just that. I am not the mom who shrieks if my boy wants to eat some junk food. In fact, I encourage it, generally choosing the unjunked junk, but on occasion, he pushes for the really bad stuff. Hey, he watches television, reads books, goes to school, has play dates, goes to parties, plays sports, and goes to camp—so exposure is inevitable.

Instead of battling with him over his intermittent bad food desires, I made the choice a while back to let him eat some of the things he begs for. Several years ago, while we were shopping at a local market, he pestered me for crushable yogurt. He said that all his friends get to eat it and that it has a cool monkey on the package. Hand in hand we walked over to the dairy aisle, and he reached for the red package.

"Mommy, p-l-e-a-s-e?" One look at the smiling monkey, and I knew the ingredient list would make me frown—high sugar, artificial flavors, and colors. I thought, *GROSS*, but to my blond-haired, brown-eyed child, I replied, "If you want to try this, you can."

He ripped open the package and started to devour the bright purple-blue foodstuff inside. Quickly coming up for air, he exclaimed, "This is disgusting, Mom!"

My kid was pissed. He went on, "How is this yogurt? Why do kids like this stuff? It's way too sweet and tastes fake." With that, he stormed over to the garbage and threw out what was left of his cup and the remaining six-pack. A valuable lesson learned—cartoon characters typically mean crappy food.

Dear readers, do you know that the fast-food and junk-food industries spend roughly $2 billion per year marketing their food to kids, whether yours or someone else's? And if the little ones watch television, they see an average of ten food-related ads per day. It doesn't stop there. Roughly six million kids ages three to eleven play some form of virtual game online each month; in 2011, food industry ad spending for this media sector was expected to reach $1 billion by 2014 (and likely more in years to come). Ninety-eight percent of the ads they see are for foods high in fat, sugar, and sodium. And might I add, these foods are packed with other gems like artificial colors and flavors and chemical preservatives.[2]

For all you caregivers out there, it is your job to provide children with a variety of healthy foods to choose from, and it is their job to decide what they will put in their mouths. That alone can be a great challenge. Now add clever food industry marketing to the mix and your job just got harder. Corporations have taken it upon themselves to tell children what is healthy with the help of character branding, whether the maniacal monkey or those darn superheroes. So any way you slice it, you are screwed.

But you do have help. First, several organizations are working to curb food marketing to children. I urge you to check these out and take action where you can: Food MythBusters (foodmyths.org); Campaign for a Commercial-Free Childhood (commercialfreechildhood.org); Corporate Accountability International (stopcorporateabuse.org); and the Center for Science in the Public Interest (cspinet.org).

CHAPTER 14

Aisle-by-Aisle Actionables

Before you hit the aisles, consider this—whether you shop at your local supermarket or at a large "natural" foods market, you will find a fair mix of healthy and not-so-healthy choices. Don't for one second think that if you buy something at a mini or mega "health food" establishment that your choice is automatically healthy. Yes, it may be devoid of most of my Top-Rated Terminators, but you should now know that when it comes to food, never judge a book by its cover.

There are other valuable tricks of the trade for navigating the nuttiness of the supermarket, all of which are based on the information already presented in this book. Fasten your seat belts and join me with your shopping cart as we ride through the aisles.

My Aisle-by-Aisle Actionables are organized from the outside of the market in. And each section, like "produce" or "frozen," has a checklist of directives called What the Fork to Do—think of it as having me talk to you while you meander through the marketplace. You can also use Appendix D, "The Practical Whole Foods Pantry," as a new blueprint for building better nourishment.

Oh, and be sure to have handy the following food and nutrition smartphone apps as they will make negotiating everything edible a little bit easier (search online and download):

1. The Environmental Working Group's (EWG) Pesticides on Produce (Dirty Dozen Plus™ and Clean 15™)
2. EWG's Food Database™

3. The Non-GMO Project's Shopping Guide and/or True Food by the Center for Food Safety
4. Animal Welfare Approved's (AWA) Food Labels Exposed
5. Monterey Bay Aquarium's Seafood Watch

On the Edge of the Market (Typically)

PRODUCE

What the Fork to Do

❑ If you can buy 100 percent organic, be my guest. In the end, this is the best way to go to reduce pesticide exposure and avoid potential GMO crops. However, if you can't find the chemical-free strawberries that you are craving, it's okay to let yourself off the hook and go for the nonorganic on occasion.

❑ If you can't buy all organic, the Dirty Dozen Plus™ and the Clean 15™ can help you navigate produce purchases. If you or anyone in your family consumes a particular fruit or vegetable *daily* that is on the Dirty Dozen Plus™ list, such as apples, then try to buy organic.

❑ Every piece of produce has a PLU (price look-up) code (though apparently it is optional for retailers). This is the way it goes:

> **Conventional Produce**—four-digit code (i.e., 4139 for Granny Smith apples)
> **Organic Produce**—five-digit code starting with a 9 (i.e., 94139 for Granny Smith apples)
> **Genetically Modified Produce**—five-digit code starting with an 8 (i.e., 84139 for Granny Smith apples), though apparently this hasn't caught on yet

❑ Buying local is my ideal (pesticides or not) because the food is at peak freshness (and also likely peak nutrition) and I like to support my local community. But if you can't go local all the time, don't shoot yourself. However, I urge you to do this—learn where your fruits and veggies come from by checking out the stickers on the food or sometimes the signage in the market. If you know the origin of your produce, then you have an idea of how long it took to travel to you. Do you really want broccoli from far away if you can get it from your farmer friend? Think about your food's footprint.

❑ If you can buy according to the seasons, then please do so. What you buy will depend on where you live regionally. The best way to do this is to join community-supported agriculture (CSA)—a way for people to buy what is in season from local farmers. This is true nourishment for you, your community, and the environment. To find a CSA near you, check out localharvest.org.

❑ While you will most likely always aim for that perfect piece of produce, love the underdogs too. In other words, if you are making an apple pie and can cut around a few small bruises, then buy the "damaged goods." Otherwise they will surely go to waste—so here's your chance to be a part of the solution versus the problem.

❑ A word to the wise about greens in a box or bag: Whatever the date, they typically go bad quickly, so buy only what you will use right away and definitely aim for those with a "use by" date as far out as possible. Heads or bunches of anything green that you can clean, strip, and rip yourself tend to keep longer.

❑ Although your greens in a clamshell may be triple washed, please give them another rinse. According to *Consumer Reports*, when triple-washed greens were tested for contamination, the bacteria found indicated poor sanitation.[1] Bottom line: You never know unless you do it yourself.

DAIRY/REFRIGERATED

What the Fork to Do

❑ This is the perfect place to pull up AWA's *Food Labels Exposed* (and refer back to chapter 11's "Decoding Marketing Madness: The Funny (and Not-So-Funny) Label Lingo"). You will see a lot of terminology like "cage free" and "hormone free" in this section and will surely need help vetting it. You can also call on the Environmental Working Group's Food Database™ to clarify some confusing ingredients.

❑ When buying dairy, whether milk or other products like butter, yogurt, and cheese, *please* try to buy organic *all the time* to limit potential antibiotic-resistant bacteria and hormone residues. Having the Animal Welfare Approved and Certified Humane labels on top of that is likely the most trustworthy combo around these days. In other words, whether your dairy says "no hormones added" or "no antibiotics" and of course "rBGH free," there is really no way to know if these labels are truthful because no form of verification exists other than my top three suggestions.

❑ If your dairy says "grassfed" with American Grassfed Association verification (and/or the Animal Welfare Approved or Food Alliance seals), then you are getting the best nutrition possible from your cow. Note that just because a product says USDA Organic noting "grass-fed," without any of the other seals it is *not* verified and likely not truly grassfed. By the way, going grassfed is superior to corn-fed cattle.

❑ For butter, ideally the ingredient list should say only "pasteurized organic sweet cream" and maybe salt. If it says "lactic acid" or "cultures," no biggie, as they are harmless and in fact part of the butter-making process. However, many butters today are packed with unnecessary additives including "natural" flavor.

❑ When you are buying the fancier cheeses, organic will be hard to come by. Give yourself a break and enjoy your gourmet goodness.

❑ As far as cheese slices (whether individually plastic wrapped or single-layered in a block are concerned), watch out because most are not really cheese, but rather processed cheese food (a cheeselike substance with other ingredients that aren't always good).

❑ Many people ask, "Why are nondairy milks in the fridge when they started out in the grocery aisle?" As more people opted for nondairy, the companies behind the liquid wanted to make the alternatives as marketable as mainstream milk. The refrigerated version is perishable (just like milk) and should be treated as such. But beware of added sugars in the many options including soy (hopefully the non-GMO variety), rice, almond, and coconut that are available today.

❑ Let's talk yogurt. Be wary of the hype, because most yogurt has tons of sugar (often diminishing yogurt's purported probiotic health benefits) and lots of flavoring even if "natural." It's best to go with the plain kind and add the sweet yourself if necessary.

❑ The advantages of Greek yogurt are many: It has about twice the protein and fewer carbs compared to regular yogurt and is thick and creamy for those who love texture. But I do suggest trying Bulgarian yogurt like Trimona—it doesn't waste the whey (the liquid part of the yogurt), as is common in Greek yogurt, and it is likely the most nutritious yogurt on the market given its probiotic profile alone.

❑ With kiddie yogurts—whether in drink, tube, or other creamy forms—watch out for the sugar, flavors, and colors regardless of the health claims.

❑ Aim for USDA Organic eggs with the AWA or Certified Humane seal of approval first. Remember, healthier animals equals a healthier you. If those aren't available, go USDA Organic alone. You can go for "cage free," "free-roaming," "pasture raised," and so on, but remember, those claims as standalones are not verified so they could very well be bogus (but perhaps a step up from conventional). Plus, don't buy into the omega hype, and eat real eggs versus the beaters.

❑ If you buy from a local farm, you can ask the producers themselves all the questions you want (and you should know what to ask by now); and you can actually see where your food, whether dairy or eggs, comes from.

❑ When you buy soy products such as tempeh (whole fermented soybeans), miso (soybean paste), and tofu (bean curd), go for the non-GMO variety.

❑ Don't think that fake bologna, or any fake meat for that matter, is better than the real deal. It is typically made from highly processed soy products with fillers and flavors. Aim for real food instead. But if mock meat is a must, then choose wisely, avoiding the TRTs.

FROZEN

What the Fork to Do

❑ EWG's Food Database™ is useful in this section as well.

❑ Keep some frozen vegetables and fruits in the freezer. Although fresh, seasonal, and local is ideal, frozen is not a bad choice. Frozen produce can actually be *more* nutritious than fresh because it's frozen soon after being picked, thus sealing nutrients into the food. And it can be less expensive than fresh. Take spinach, for example: A container of organic fresh spinach (I buy only organic here because spinach is one of the top contenders on the Dirty Dozen Plus™) is anywhere from $4 to $6. When cooked, it yields about ¾ cup of wilted spinach. A box of organic frozen spinach is anywhere from $2 to $3 and when cooked yields roughly 1½ cups. So what do you think is the better deal?

❑ Speaking of seasonal, bring on the berries during off-season in frozen form. They are great for smoothies and much more nutritious than their typically unseasonal and imported counterparts.

❑ Frozen sprouted breads are fabulous as they are packed with vital nutrition (they are kept in the freezer because they spoil more quickly than their shelf-stable counterparts). So definitely dabble in these breads and keep them in the fridge once opened to prevent spoiling.

❑ Don't let prepared frozen foods woo you too much. They are typically loaded with extra sodium, sugar, and fat. However, there are some great brands out there, like Amy's, that have reduced-sodium versions. And they are quite tasty.

❑ While you may think that the veggie burger is the healthy way to satiate your "Big Mac attack," most veggie patties are highly processed and quite junky (GMO soy being a choice ingredient). Look for the burger with the fewest ingredients. Sunshine is my favorite choice.

❑ Ice cream is ice cream. It is ideal to buy organic because you want ice cream from the undrugged cow, but it's hard to come by. Choose the one you like (with the fewest and least-offensive ingredients) and stick with it. Or try out some dairy-free options made from rice milk, non-GMO soy milk, or coconut milk. And don't forget succulent sorbet and *real* fruit ice pops. Oh, and watch out for artificial sweeteners here, as they absolutely abound in frozen delights.

MEAT, POULTRY, AND SEAFOOD

What the Fork to Do

❑ You definitely want guidance with AWA's Food Labels Exposed and Seafood Watch's smartphone apps for anything fleshy.

❑ Sadly, when buying any kind of meat, pork, or poultry product today, you can't trust much. Roughly 97 percent of all U.S. meats (and even some organics) are from CAFOs. So your best bet is to aim for USDA organic with the added value of the AWA or Certified Humane seals of approval (the highest level of animal welfare is ensured). Organic alone is okay, and American Humane Certified could perhaps make a small difference. Next up, although not verified, should be "hormone free" and "antibiotic free" and some of the other semiuseful (yet possibly bogus) terms listed in AWA's guide or Chapter 11's section "Decoding Marketing Madness: The Funny (and Not-So-Funny) Label Lingo." If you are utterly discouraged about animal foods, I get it. Check out animalwelfareapproved.org or certifiedhumane.org, and you can buy your meat online from a certified farmer.

❑ Your local farmer who is doing the right thing (even without these added certifications) could be another great choice. If you visit the meadow and talk to the people in charge, you will get all the info you need (again, you should know the right questions to ask by now).

❏ You really can't trust any animal food (especially nonorganic) adorned with terms like "no hormones added," "no antibiotics," "no animal by-products," "vegetarian-fed," or others as standalones (meaning *not* accompanied by humane/high-welfare certification or organic), because there is no *real* verification for these claims.

❏ Grassfed is the way to go for the health and well-being of the cattle and you. True verification comes from the American Grassfed Association. Animal Welfare Approved (AWA) is top-notch too and look out for Food Alliance (FA). If your product says "grassfed" without any of these seals, not-so-quietly question it.

❏ Seventy percent of ground beef products contain lean finely textured beef (LFTB), better known as "pink slime." This totally unsavory filler is composed of low-grade beef trimmings, cartilage, tendons, and connective tissue that is heated and treated with gaseous ammonia to kill bacteria and is then pressed into pellets and used as a filler in your beef. According to the USDA, LFTB is considered beef so it does not have to be identified as an ingredient in ground beef. One by one, stores are nixing their beef with pink slime, but the best way to ensure that you are really eating 100 percent unslimed beef is to opt out of the more mainstream choices, or better yet, watch your butcher grind it.

❏ For seafood, it is imperative to have Seafood Watch handy when trying to understand your best consumption options.

❏ The hard truth about your fish and shellfish (as noted in sidebar, "A Fishy Situation" on page 80) is that roughly 91 percent of seafood in the United States is imported, and with that comes a cycle of freezing and thawing, chemical preservation, and filth. If you can't find truly local fish (as in you know the boat or person who caught it, or at least your vendor knows them), look for the Country of Origin Labeling (COOL) to see if it came from the United States. Aim to choose truly local friends from the sea that go from Dock to Dish.

❏ Is your fish "wild"? If so, from where and what was its journey to get to you? If from aquaculture, is the farm copacetic? Your best bet is seafood raised in a closed recirculating farm (meaning an on-land closed-loop system where waste and water are reused and recycled). Be sure to ask your fishmonger questions or, better yet, when it comes to farms, do a little research.

❏ Then there is contamination—according to the Natural Resources Defense Council, the fish highest in mercury are mackerel (king), marlin, orange roughy, shark, swordfish, tilefish, and tuna (bigeye, ahi). Other fish with high levels are bluefish, grouper, mackerel (Spanish, gulf), sea bass (Chilean), and tuna (canned albacore, yellowfin). Given the mercury in these fish, consumption should be limited to weekly, even monthly (and sometimes not at all), especially for pregnant women and young children. The NRDC sheds further light on this issue and has a mercury calculator to boot: nrdc.org/health/effects/mercury/guide.asp.[2] Also, to stay updated and informed on all other fish matters, check in with Seafood Watch.

❏ Do you love the fish that is on its way to extinction or is being fished in an unsustainable fashion? Seafood Watch can help you here too.

❏ Salmon and Arctic char turn pink in the wild because they naturally consume shrimp (giving them their pink-red hue). When farmed, both fish are often given dyes in their feed (whether from a natural source like beta-carotene or a synthetic one such as Red Dye No. 40). Stick with wild salmon or know the practices of your farm.

❏ On seafood identity, a 2013 study from Oceana, a sea-loving conservation group, revealed that roughly one third of the fish you eat is mislabeled. In other words, your cod can be tilapia, and so can your snapper. So be sure to ask questions.

❏ My seafood ideal is my local community-supported fishery (CSF) called Dock to Dish. As a member, I receive a weekly share of fish directly from the fishermen in my community. You can't beat that. If you live in a coastal community, is there a CSF in your vicinity? Check out localcatch.org to find out. Or buy from your local fishmonger, who sources directly from the boats.

❑ If you can't go local, buy with your eyes wide open, knowing that your fish has most likely traveled quite a distance to get to you. And more often than not, it has already been frozen to keep it "fresh." But as far as overall nutrition is concerned, a little fish can be better than none. And don't forget that frozen, if caught and processed in the United States, is the best non-local great alternative.

❑ As far as fish and preservatives are concerned, sulfites should be labeled if above 10 ppm (parts per million). Sodium tripolyphosphate (STPP) will most likely not be labeled, but ask if your fish (primarily shrimp and scallops) are "wet" (meaning they were soaked). Make sure you go for the "dry" version. In general, don't be shy to ask if chemicals were used in any way. Cross your fingers for the truth.

❑ When buying shellfish, like oysters, mussels, and clams, look for hand collected, raked, or rope or bag grown.

❑ On organic fish, Food and Water Watch has this to say: "Currently, there is no U.S. government-approved organic seafood. These products are often labeled as organic based on criteria set by a private certification company, or in accord with European standards. Neither of these usually equate to U.S. organic standards for other foods."[3] In other words, there is really no such thing as organic seafood.

❑ AquaAdvantage Salmon (the GMO variety) may very well be in the marketplace compliments of AquaBounty Technologies. And there is no way for you to know if your pink-fleshed finfish has been genetically altered—the FDA does not require labeling. In March 2014, nine thousand stores across the country rejected this salmon. So just be sure to do a little recon with your fishmonger about this frankenfish.

DELI/PREPARED FOODS

What the Fork to Do

❑ Be wary of any lunch meat (whether "freshly" sliced, dogs, jerky, or bacon) with added nitrates and nitrites, as the safety of these chemicals is questionable. There are many choices today like Applegate that are free of these added synthetics.

❏ Whether sliced ham or hot dogs, these "choice" meats typically come with fillers—everything from sugar to flour, fibers, flavors, and more.

❏ When choosing cured foods, whether salmon or meats, which are preserved by either smoking or adding sugar, salt, or nitrates/nitrites (try to avoid these), you want to know if the food was naturally smoked (exposed to burning or smoldering plant materials such as wood) or if fake flavor was added. Typically, the latter is the case. If the meat was preserved with additives, were synthetic chemicals or simply sugar or salt used?

❏ If you are purchasing prepared foods, give them a good glance and even ask for a taste, as they may not be as fresh as they seem. A word to the wise: Be wary of buying prepared foods at the end of the day. Chances are that they have been sitting around in the viewing case, under lights, and manhandled all day.

❏ Always question the sanitation of a salad bar. While you may be able to trust the store and the sneeze guard, you *can't* truly trust the many people who frequent the food. And when dressing your salad, aim for the oil and vinegar rather than the bottles of flavor that are most likely laced with TRTs.

BAKERY

What the Fork to Do

❏ Commercially baked goods are typically trans fat culprits. Since the FDA is trying to rid your food supply of trans fats, man-made vegetable oils are most likely being replaced with palm or coconut oil. Yes, these are better for your health, but note that although both come from plants, they are high in saturated fat. And if you overconsume them, you could surely suffer. So enjoy the sporadic baked good.

❑ Question the ingredients on all baked goods, even if they are "fresh," because many soft, chewy delights may not be as healthy as they seem, meaning that a bran muffin may be no different from its chocolate chip counterpart in sugar content and more.

❑ Is the baking done on the premises or is it done in a factory far off? Not that this makes a difference in ingredients, but it can affect freshness.

On the Inside of the Market (Typically)

BAKING AISLE

What the Fork to Do

❑ Watch out for the bleached enriched flours—remember that they have been touched by chemicals and enhanced with nutrition to renourish. Aim for the unbleached, less refined flours such as "whole wheat" (with the Whole Grain seal of approval) with the sustenance sealed in.

❑ Pick and choose baking mixes wisely. Most are muddled with tons of TRTs.

❑ When buying extracts, aim for those that are *real* versus the imitation flavoring sort.

❑ Baking powders and sodas are pretty pure as is.

❑ No matter what sugar you choose (whether granulated or liquid), please go for the real stuff as opposed to the bag or bottle of fake. And steer clear of the syrupy corn.

❑ When choosing maple syrup, again go for the 100 percent pure maple. Also note that the syrups are graded based on translucence. Maple with an A (whether light amber, also known as "fancy"; medium amber; or dark amber) means it's lighter in color; maple with a B means it's darker in color (and typically richer in flavor).

❑ Most frostings, icings, and decorations like anything sprinkly (plus those little bottles of green, yellow, red, and blue) are loaded with TRTs such as artificial colors and flavors. But there are better options, and you will find them in Appendix B, "Common Food Brands and Recommended Alternatives."

❑ If buying anything chocolatey and chippy, keep watch for those with artificial flavoring.

Boasting BPA-Free

BPA, or bisphenol A, is a chemical that has been used to make certain plastics since the 1960s. Typically found in polycarbonate form, which is moldable when exposed to heat, it is a common component of containers that store your food and beverages—for example, as a coating for the interior of cans, or the material used for any bottle or edible repository. It is thought to be an endocrine disrupter by the National Institutes of Health: "Endocrine disruptors are chemicals that may interfere with the body's endocrine system and produce adverse developmental, reproductive, neurological, and immune effects in both humans and wildlife."[4] According to the FDA, which stood by BPA until 2010, "Studies employing standardized toxicity tests have thus far supported the safety of current low levels of human exposure to BPA. However, on the basis of results from recent studies using novel approaches to test for subtle effects, both the National Toxicology Program at the National Institutes of Health and FDA has some concern about the potential effects of BPA on the brain, behavior, and prostate gland in fetuses, infants, and young children."[5]

Nonetheless, the FDA has *not* issued a cease-and-desist on BPA. Rather, "in cooperation with the National Toxicology Program, FDA's National Center for Toxicological Research is carrying out in-depth studies to answer key questions and clarify uncertainties about the risks of BPA." As a consequence, many companies now boast BPA-free containers, and some companies have opted out of using them in cans. I suggest that you do your best to avoid anything BPA. On the bottom of most plastic containers is a recycling code—7 means that the plastic most likely contains BPA (so you want to avoid it); 3 and 6 are somewhat unsavory as well, containing other endocrine-disrupting chemicals. The safer choices are 1, 2, 4, and 5.

To learn more about BPA and other endocrine disrupting chemicals (some of which are already mentioned in this book) visit ewg.org to download a copy of their *Dirty Dozen™ List of Endocrine Disruptors—12 Hormone Altering Chemicals and How to Avoid Them.*

CANNED, BOXED, BOTTLED, AND BAGGED

What the Fork to Do

- ❑ You definitely want the Environmental Working Group's Food Database™ and the Non-GMO Project's Shopping Guide (or True Food by the Center for Food Safety) at your fingertips for this section.
- ❑ Big Food is vying for prime shelf space; thus it is highly likely that at your little loved ones' eye level will be foods endorsed by superheroes and filled with TRTs. Be prepared for the pestering and hold strong to the healthy.
- ❑ Whether canned, boxed, bottled, or bagged, your food is likely infested with TRTs. So investigate ingredients here.
- ❑ If you can't pronounce an ingredient, it's probably a chemical that is not worth consuming.
- ❑ If you frequent fat-free, think twice as the fat is replaced with sugar (or even fake sugar) and its many euphemisms. And the sugar (which is often overabundant) inevitably turns into fat once eaten. So you are better with real fat from the get-go.
- ❑ "Low sugar," "reduced sugar," "no added sugar," "zero calories," or "calorie-free" can mean that your food is typically sweetened with the artificials.

❏ In general, watch out for sugar and salt content in anything packaged—it is customarily quite high.

❏ Processed foods typically gloat about their goodness, whether they claim to be high fiber, high protein, or rich in antioxidants, vitamins, and minerals. Don't be fooled—much of the nutrition is stripped away during processing and then added back in. Don't buy into health claims, please, whether these or any others.

❏ Are your herbs and spices irradiated? If they are organic, presume that they are *not* irradiated. A handful of aromatic makers, such as Frontier, ensure that their products are non-irradiated. If you don't see that term on your jar of herb or spice, presume it was zapped.

❏ When buying spice mixes, bouillons, and broths, keep an eye out for TRTs and MSG, and of course note that irradiation is most likely inevitable.

❏ When considering large containers of bargain ground herbs and spices, question whether they are adulterated. Chances are that they could be. Stick with the smaller jars and reputable brand names such as Frontier and McCormick.

❏ When buying oils, try not to buy into the bargains because most likely the liquid is inferior or laced with GMO canola, cottonseed, or soy. Avoid "light" because it really means nothing (other than "no nutrition").

❏ You are typically safe when buying vinegars, tomato sauce, olives, and sauerkraut, but definitely don't skip the ingredient lists. You can never be too sure.

❏ Watch out for the toxic yellow dye in pickles, relishes, and similar condiments. It is totally unnecessary, and better options abound.

❏ For animal foods in a tin (even seafood), buyer beware. They are often loaded with salt and some notoriously nasty TRTs (and highly unlikely to be high welfare).

❏ Select soups wisely since many are loaded with sodium, MSG, and other TRTs. And try to find cans without BPA. Some do exist. Better yet, buy the soups in a glass jar or box.

❏ For grains in a box, whether pasta (like mac and cheese) or seasoned grain mixes, don't dig in for nutrition because it's really not there. Pick and choose wisely, watching out for TRTs, or go for real whole-grain goodness.

❏ Beans are best without added chemicals; they do just fine with a little added salt. Note that baked beans can boast unnecessary sugar. Keep a lookout and try to buy BPA-free packaging.

❏ For anything sugary, from jam to maple syrup, go for the real deal rather than the imitation variety.

❏ Applesauce *does not* need added sugar.

❏ Most nutty butters have added oil (often the GMO variety) and sugar. Straight up is the healthiest way to go. If you need a little sweet to take the edge off, plenty of options on the market are slightly sweet (using a touch of honey or even sugar) versus the all-too-common over-sugared choices.

SNACKS

What the Fork to Do

❏ Snack foods, whether crackers, chips, pretzels, or crunchy cheesy bites, love trans fats. As these hydrogenated oils are being phased out as per the FDA, they are being replaced with good vegetable oil in the form of palm or coconut (though both are high in saturated fat). Be careful of overconsumption—not only will your animal foods have saturated fat, but your processed foods will too.

❏ Lots of crunch, especially the flavored chips, contain crap. Most often they are laced with fake color and flavor.

❏ Many snacks today boast function (as in high protein, high fiber) and less evil. Folks, please don't consider any crunch a viable delivery system for nutrition. Eat them for pleasure, not health. And anything other than a plain potato chip or simple corn chip is overly processed, so pick and choose wisely—whether "healthy" or not.

Energy Bars—The Glorified Candy Bar

Most bars (granola, power, energy, meal replacement, etc.) are doppel-gängers for the candy kind. They are packed with sugar (and its many euphemisms, whether brown rice syrup, barley malt, or cane sugar); highly processed protein as in soy protein isolates; manufactured crunch; and chocolate (typically not the good dark kind). The added value? The oodles of vitamins and minerals that are dumped in to make you think that you are eating something super healthy . . .

Think again. If you want a bar that boosts, go for the real food kind comprised of nuts, seeds, dried fruit, dark chocolate, and even a little sugar. Avoid the highly processed protein, insane amounts of added nutrients, and those with ingredient lists that read like a short novel. I urge you to check out my top choices when it comes to bars of any sort of bounty:

- Bumble Bar
- Oskri
- The Pure Bar
- Health Warrior Chia Bars
- Kate's Real Food Bars
- Kind Bar (though watch out for some of their powerful protein varieties)

You can even build your own bar at youbars.com, or better yet, how about a Do-It-Yourself grab-and-go trail mix (without the added sugared fruit and candy) that will give you all you need for a wholesome pick-me-up during the day.

BEVERAGES

What the Fork to Do

❑ Other than flat and carbonated water and truly unsweetened beverages like tea, most bottled liquid is loaded with sugar and other TRTs, so undoubtedly analyze.

❑ Speaking of tea, many ready-to-drink teas come from tea extracted from tea leaves, which is then processed with chemicals (albeit possibly "natural" chemicals) to enhance stability, color, and other properties, then spray-dried with a food starch (most likely maltodextrin from GMO corn), then further mixed and manipulated to taste like tea. In the end, is this really tea? I don't think so. Sadly, even the companies that rave about their realness are not all that. Thus, examine—meaning give the company a call to question their brewing process (or even if they brew it at all).

❑ If you go for the juice in the fridge, whether orange or grapefruit, note that "not from concentrate" means that the juice was freshly squeezed from the fruit itself and pasteurized, and neither water, sugar, nor preservatives were added. On the other hand, "from concentrate" means that the juice was extracted from the fruit and the water was removed, forming a rich mixture for future reconstitution with water. Either way, both can be enhanced with nutrients. In the end, don't seek nutrition from the sweet sauce (unless it is being squeezed by hand in your presence).

❑ Liquid lemon and lime juice, more often than not, is neither pure nor real (despite claims to the contrary). So just buy the citrus and squeeze yourself.

❑ Be wary of hidden sulfites in citrus concentrates. Oftentimes the added citric acid, when processed, is treated with sulfuric acid, leaving sulfite residues behind (albeit below the 10 ppm).

❑ Smoothies in a small bottle sporting health bravado should be scrutinized. Most are loaded with sugar (whether from the fruit or added sweetness) and processed protein (if it's pushing the "pump") and honestly don't deliver much real nutrition. In a pinch they are okay, but otherwise find the fresh.

❑ In anything diet, the superficial sweetness that you think is your best friend may very well be your worst enemy. Try not to drink dangerously—how about some bubbly water with a splash of juice or squeeze of citrus?

❑ When buying shelf-stable nondairy milks (or any milk, for that matter), pick what you like, but know that many are spiked with some form of sugar. Go for the unsweetened and think of milk as a condiment (whether in coffee, tea, or cereal) rather than a stein of sustenance.

❑ If you do decaffeinated, understand that anything naturally containing caffeine (such as coffee, black tea, or green tea) is typically treated in some way to remove the caffeine, which can involve everything from water to synthetic chemicals. It's good to be in the know.

❑ Energy-boosting drinks are pretty scary stuff. They are often loaded with inordinate amounts of caffeine—anywhere from 50 to 2,100 mg (or more!) per 8 ounces, which is seriously almost enough to race a horse's heart, not to mention that some other choice TRTs are present as well.

On Bottled Water

For drinking water on the go, I urge people to go green, meaning get yourself a stainless steel bottle like a good old Klean Kanteen (kleankanteen.com) or a BPA-free canister for use and reuse. They are durable and more affordable than buying "plastic water" day in and day out.

According to the Natural Resources Defense Council, bottled water may very well be a total bust:

"NRDC conducted a four-year review of the bottled water industry and the safety standards that govern it, including a comparison of national bottled water rules with national tap water rules, and independent testing of over 1,000 bottles of water. Our conclusion is that there is no assurance that just because water comes out of a bottle it is any cleaner or safer than water from the tap. And in fact, an estimated 25 percent or more of bottled water is really just tap water in a bottle—sometimes further treated, sometimes not."[6]

And to add insult to injury, the environmental, physical, and economic consequences of gulping water in a disposable bottle are staggering. The water experts at GRACE Communications Foundation had this to offer from *Why You Should Never Buy Disposable Water Bottles Again* (greatist.com). Here are a few facts to whet your appetite:

- Even though the United States has some of the safest tap water in the world, it has the largest market for bottled water—roughly 30 billion bottles per year.
- Bottled water costs three hundred to two thousand times more than tap water.
- Drinking eight glasses of tap water per day costs roughly $0.50/year while the same consumption of bottled water costs about $1,400/year.
- More than 80 percent of water bottles end up in landfills (while some are recycled, many also end up littering roadsides and waterways).[7]

Not only is bottled water a total bust (though perhaps necessary at times), but it also clearly causes avoidable environmental suffering. And should you opt out, it will surely add dollars to your pocket. Your best bet is to Take Back the Tap (in a reusable bottle) by visiting foodandwaterwatch.org/water/take-back-the-tap/.

CHAPTER 15

Strategies for Introducing New Nourishment

(for Kids and Grown-ups)

Let's face it—the most difficult part of your task is not going to be clearing out your pantry and checking labels one by one. If you are reading *What the Fork*, you are motivated on some level. The toughest part will far and away be convincing your family to get on board. So you have to make it fun while also setting some new boundaries and ground rules.

Talk to the adults about what you plan to do for you and your kids (if you have them) and hand them a copy of this book, but in the end they will make their own choices. Kids (from birth onward) develop healthy eating habits by modeling grown-ups. Thus constant exposure to healthy food and conversation about food is critical. Before suggesting some tested get-on-board strategies, I would like to establish a few ground rules:

1. Never presume your child (or even your partner/spouse) won't like something. I bet you are already thinking that you won't buy this or that because you know that they won't like it. If you have an open mind, it's likely that they will too.
2. Make a rule that everyone has to try something *once*.
3. Never quit on introducing new foods. If your kid (or resident grown-up) doesn't like the new Better for You Alternative of those chocolate sandwich cookies, keep reintroducing. For fresh

food like broccoli, relentlessly reintroduce (at two-week intervals), but think about how you are preparing it (perhaps you
should sauté it with some olive oil, even add a little butter, rather
than steam it, or try Skillet Broccoli on page 256).

4. When your child does not like a food, talk to them about why
they don't like it. Explain to them why it is healthy. For example,
"Spinach can give you muscles like your professional athlete
hero . . ."

5. Never forget that it is your job as a caregiver to provide your children with a variety of healthy foods, and it is their job to choose
what to eat within that context. If they skip a meal, they won't
starve.

6. Don't push food on your kids (as in "you must eat everything on
your plate"); children need to learn how to self-regulate.

Supermarket Scavenger Hunt

Kids can be a hindrance while food shopping for sure. So how about making them an asset? You can give older children a list of food items to find
and send them on a Supermarket Scavenger Hunt (with their own cart
and all). You will not only be orienting them toward the grocery shopping experience (a good tool to have for self-sufficiency later in life) but
also guiding them toward better food choices. As in any scavenger hunt,
there can be a prize of some sort at the end of the "game" (the chance to
pick a healthy treat, or perhaps a trip to the movies with a friend).

Those who are too little to scavenge on their own can hunt with you by
their side. Create a list and ask them to identify each item as you stroll
through the aisles. Reward them accordingly as suggested earlier. This ends
up being fun for the kids no matter the age and helpful for you.

The Taste-Testing Experiment

The Taste-Testing Experiment is a great activity to do with your kids (and even your partner/spouse) to get them involved and make it a little easier for them to give up their not-so-healthy choices. Using your Reaper Rescue Guide (from chapter 13) as a starting point, select two healthier alternatives for that food at the grocery store (use Appendix B, "Common Food Brands and Recommended Alternatives" to help here) and set up a taste test at home. For example, the fabulous fruit roll-up's Better for You Alternative can be found in Stretch Island's FruitaBü or even their fruit leather. To get your kids into the spirit of the "test," blindfold them if you have to. And let them taste the Grim Reaper and the Better for You Alternative. Then talk about the experience with them. Odds are good that once they try the healthier but just as yummy choices, they'll be open to trying more of the Keepers.

The Arts and Crafts Kitchen

My son Hunter is extraordinarily picky (see sidebar, "Respecting Funny Little Eating Habits," page 212). So to ease his pain and mine, I turned to what I do best—cooking. He has gone from the kid who eats nothing to the kid who loves to cook, eats what he cooks, and is now more open to trying new things (a huge step).

Most kids' palates expand when they are allowed to touch and taste anything edible. Think arts and crafts but with food. While it may be more stressful for you, it's worthwhile to bear it with a smile on your face. So I urge you to get the kids touching and playing with edibles at an early age (as soon as they can sit in a high chair). This can then evolve into cooking with them. With a kitchen stool, a butter knife, a cutting board, and some soft foods to get started (such as mushrooms and cheese), your kids will be little cooks in no time. One of my favorite go-to resources for all things kid-and-cooking-related is julienegrin.com.

Respecting Funny Little Eating Habits

My younger son was born with feeding issues. I am thrilled to know that the powers that be have a sense of humor.

Shortly after Hunter was born, my sweet husband remained with him while the nurses did their necessary newborn testing in the nursery. As I was in and out of sleep, my man, with our little guy and the nurse in tow, came into the room to tell me, "Hunter's tongue is heart shaped."

How cute, my boy had a heart-shaped tongue. Then the nurse chimed in, "It seems that your son is tongue-tied. I am not sure how this will affect his feeding, but I would like his doctor to take a look."

Fear swept over me, but I tried to rationalize it: *He has ten fingers and ten toes. Feeding issues I can deal with.* The doctor arrived to confirm that Hunter had a congenital oral anomaly that might affect his ability to eat, but we wouldn't know anything for a few days. The worst-case scenario would be if he had to have the membrane connecting the underside of his tongue with the floor of his mouth (frenulum) cut by a specialist. Pretty gnarly, but what could we do?

As it turned out, Hunter couldn't eat. Whether breast milk or formula, it would pour out of his mouth. He lost weight daily, so at our pediatrician's demand, we brought him to a specialist at seven days old to get clipped. Thinking his tongue was released so he would finally be able to eat, we let out a huge sigh of relief.

But that was not the case. After the frenulectomy (the clinical term for tongue snipping), it took him more than an hour to drink 3 ounces from a bottle (I couldn't breast-feed for long due to personal medical issues); for reference, most newborns can down that in ten to fifteen minutes. He was miserable, and so were we. So we went back to the pediatrician and learned that he had a condition called hypotonia (low muscle tone) in his facial muscles, and as a result, he had difficulty coordinating sucking and swallowing. Then we were off to the swallowing therapist twice weekly for nine months to learn how to improve Hunter's facial muscle tone so he could eat, and manage this arduous and highly emotional journey with our son. Not an easy task.

So the culinary nutritionist who knows how to help solve others' food problems couldn't help her own son. I had to learn how to be okay with the fact that Hunter's *main source of nourishment* was from the bottle long after the average age of six to eight months (the "typical" age at which a child begins to transition to solid foods)—once he learned how to suck, he didn't want to stop. And when he finally did take solids, he gagged and threw up until he was just over a year old. If you touched what was on his plate, he would throw it all on the floor, and feeding time was officially over—he liked control. When he finally did start to eat more regularly (around eighteen months), his menu was highly limited—pasta and chicken were about as far as I could take him.

But I never gave up. I followed his lead and kept introducing and reintroducing foods until he tried them, always letting him feel like he had some level of control. I talked to him about food, took him food shopping, and surrendered to him as my regular sidekick in the kitchen (not an easy task). My little one had been through quite a bit, and I wanted to honor how he needed to do things.

So when clients come to me wanting me to fix their child's picky eating habits, I always aim to understand why eating is an issue. I have learned to respect funny little eating habits because you never know what a child's journey truly is. As for Hunter, his medical condition shaped his initial relationship with food—not a good one. And it was and still is my job to guide him toward a connection with food that will keep him safe and healthy through life.

The *Chopped* Competition

Have you ever watched *Chopped* on the Food Network? Picture this: four chefs, a basket of four obscure ingredients, and the task of creating a dish within a fairly short time frame. There are three rounds, and at the end of each, a chef is eliminated, finally leaving one as the winner of $10,000.

Now, I am not a big TV watcher, but this show surely planted a seed in my already overactive mind as I watched it with my boys. We created a family version of *Chopped*. My husband bought the ingredients (scallops, red potatoes, cucumber, and pineapple), and Jack and I competed (though we didn't set a time limit—a much safer way to do it with kids) while Hunter watched and eventually made a concoction of his own. We had a blast and it was a great way for me to connect with my boys around food. This is what we came up with:

1. Jack—Scallop soup; seared scallops with pan-fried diced potatoes; cucumber spears and sliced pineapple
2. Me—Seared scallops over potato hash with a grilled-pineapple-and-cucumber salsa

In the end, we not only cooked but also chatted about ingredients, meal preparation, and our creations and shared a meal together as a family. But most important, Hunter, my picky child who prefers food from a box, ate fish and mushrooms for the very first time! Everyone was on board that evening.

Show It and Say It on Social Media

I had just *unwillingly* (I wouldn't call myself incredibly social-media savvy) launched a Pinterest board, when one day, while cooking and posting, I caught Jack, then six, peering over my shoulder, "Hey, Mom, can I do one of those?"

It was the birth of an idea—we started a board, "Jack Loves Food," where we posted photos from our many food adventures whether shopping or cooking. Since, we have put Pinterest aside for Facebook, Instagram, and the fabulous Feedfeed (feedfeed.info), a social media platform (and smartphone app) that is 100 percent food-centric—connecting people all over the world on everything edible from inspiration to actual recipes. You can find me on all three under "Stefanie Sacks" (I am finally getting better at social media), and know that many of the photos are compliments of Jack and his little brother, Hunter, as we love to take pics of anything food related and share the nourishment. Actively posting together has been a great way to keep the conversation going, and I urge you to try it with your little ones.

Don't Judge a Book by Its Cover

If your kid or even your spouse is *seriously hooked* on a food with TRTs, opt for the Better for You Alternative. For example, you can swap the Ritz crackers for Barbara's Rite Rounds. But instead of offering the Rite Rounds straight up, packaging and all, remove the American staple from its box and fill it with the better brand. I know, it's a little sneaky, but I have seen it work. When your eater says, "Hmmm, these taste a little different," assuming they do, just reply with, "Perhaps the company has just enhanced their product." It may sound like a long shot, but I swear it is worth a try. Then, when Barbara's has comfortably made its way into your pantry, you can do a big reveal with your picky eater. But do your best not to revert to the Grim Reaper.

Moving on from the "Meat" of the Makeover

Hopefully you feel a tad more educated (and perhaps a little entertained). I realize that you are probably on information overload, but hold close to your heart that any change, no matter how small, can make big everyday differences. Now come with me to *realistically* rehab your meals and to get cooking.

Meal Rehab

If I could buy 100 percent organic, I would, across the board. I relish farm stands, farmers markets, and health food stores. I like to buy my meats from the person who's raising them right and fish from my local fisherman. But that is just *not* my reality all the time. And quite honestly, it is not many people's reality. So my job is to teach people how to work with what they *have*, what they *can do*, what they are *willing to do*, and what *makes sense* for them, while at the same time *helping them do a little better so they can be as healthy as possible.*

My intention is *not* to shove chia seeds or tempeh down the throats of America, or persuade you to eat raw foods versus cooked food. My plan is to offer as much guidance as possible for planning meals and preparing some serious yum. Let's face it: At this point you should know (or at least have an idea of) how to procure anything edible.

This is the deal: I am not here to aid weight loss—that's for the good old diet books. However, according to the Centers for Disease Control, fad diets limit your nutritional intake, can be unhealthy, and tend to fail in the long run. Go figure. It's all about your food lifestyle (that's what I like to call this whole transition), and that's what I aim to shift here by teaching you how to balance your plate (including a little planning advice) and getting your butt in the kitchen.

What do you need to know? Your plate will never be balanced—that means consuming healthy, wholesome food and beverages for regular meals and snacks throughout the day—if you don't know what is off kilter in the first place. So let's take a magnifying glass to what you are *really* eating and how you are doing so. And while you are busy balancing and then cooking, you may very well, in the end, lose weight. Though I won't make any promises.

CHAPTER 16

Balancing Your Plate

Shifting your food lifestyle begins with understanding what (and how) you are currently eating, identifying the problems or obstacles that are preventing you from eating healthfully, and determining what you can do about it. So let's consider this an action chapter—your essential workbook that will help you understand your relationship with food on many levels and how you can begin changing.

In a not-so-recent conversation with my rock-star friend, who is notorious for her elaborate party preparations, her beach cooler creations (for days at the ocean with the kids), and doing her best to nourish her three little ones, she confessed that her own eats are often subpar. I was slightly mortified to find out that on her way to and from gigs, she jets into a bright-light convenience mart to grab some whatever-you-want-to-call-it. Her health and well-being are super important to me. Just as yours are.

If she has time to plan and cook for the party and beach feast and nourish her kids, why can't she find a moment to take care of herself, the caregiver? Sometimes people just need a little help shifting priorities. And often the solution is very simple: planning ahead.

So this is the advice I gave my friend to organize eats for herself and her family:

1. On a Friday or over the course of the weekend (or whatever day best suits you), take ten to fifteen minutes to plan a menu for the upcoming week.

2. Then take a minute to look at your upcoming week's schedule to determine when you will be able to food shop and cook.

3. For food shopping, I like to do a *big* shop once or twice a month with a smaller shop weekly as perishables are needed; this tactic is useful if you want to save time and money and limit food waste. And, of course, I have my CSA and CSF (Dock to Dish) is season.

4. Even as an avid cook, I can't be in the kitchen every night, so I aim to cook three nights per week.

5. For the other nights, I pick a day during the week to prepare a few staple dishes such as vegetarian chili, turkey meatballs, and a soup or two (all resident recipes in this book). This helps guarantee Stefanie-approved nourishment on the nights that I can't cook. With a little reheating and supplementation with a quick salad, vegetable, and/or starch, a balanced meal is born.

6. And there are those nights that pizza or some prepared food is what feeds the frenzy.

My reality is not different from most. Navigating food is just my expertise. So take some advice from this soul sister: Planning food for you and your family a week in advance will save you time and money and reduce stress. Create realistic goals for yourself, even if it means that you cook only one or two nights per week. For many, that alone is a great start.

But there is more to balancing your plate than just planning. Remember, food choice is a deep-rooted issue and one that will not change overnight. To help my clients shift, I work with a tried and tested methodology that helps them view their relationship with food from a different veranda. And it begins with a *food diary*, followed by a *plan of action* and a little insight into the What the Fork *food philosophy* (much of which you have gleaned from this book already). We eventually end up in the kitchen, where my clients learn how to nourish themselves and have a blast doing it with me by their side.

What the Fork Food Diary

Most of the people I have worked with over the years, regardless of socio-economic status, are utterly disconnected from the food they put into their mouths. Most *swear* that they know exactly what they eat each day (and yes, many do know), but most have no idea *how* they are eating. Do you opt out of breakfast? Do you skip meals or leave more than three hours between eats? Are you a late-night binger? How much alcohol do you really drink?

To help a client, I need to know not only what they are eating but also *how* they are eating; thus I always ask each person to keep a one-week food diary. More often than not, clients say, "Seriously, Stefanie, a freakin' food diary?"

My reply: "I won't know what to fix if I can't find out what's broken." This is an exercise in conscious eating, and each person must eat as they normally do while keeping a food diary (meaning, don't try to impress). A food diary is a way to collect data points: (1) when you are eating, (2) what you are choosing to eat, and (3) how you feel after each meal or snack. With this information, mapping out how to help someone make small (and sometimes large), critical (and realistic) changes to improve their overall relationship with food is possible.

Even after their exasperated initial reaction, believe it or not, 99 percent of all people asked to keep the "freakin' food diary" do so. And 100 percent of these people come back with some form of, "I can't believe how much (or how little) I eat," "I never realized that I drink so many sugary beverages," "I had no idea that I eat so many sweets," "I didn't realize that I go four to six hours without eating," or "I didn't realize I drink that much alcohol."

Well, folks, now it is your turn. While I can't be there to review all of your diaries, simply recording what you eat for five to seven days will help you see what is broken. And once you can see where the "weakness" lies, shifting can begin with the guidance from *What the Fork* and a little promise on your part. If you are reading this book, you are ready for some form of change. So let's get a move on.

DAY ONE

MEAL	TIME	FOOD/ BEVERAGE INTAKE	HOW DO YOU FEEL (tired, bloated, hungry, etc.)
BREAKFAST			
SNACK			
LUNCH			
SNACK			
DINNER			
SNACK			

DAY TWO

MEAL	TIME	FOOD/ BEVERAGE INTAKE	HOW DO YOU FEEL (tired, bloated, hungry, etc.)
BREAKFAST			
SNACK			
LUNCH			
SNACK			
DINNER			
SNACK			

DAY THREE

MEAL	TIME	FOOD/ BEVERAGE INTAKE	HOW DO YOU FEEL (tired, bloated, hungry, etc.)
BREAKFAST			
SNACK			
LUNCH			
SNACK			
DINNER			
SNACK			

DAY FOUR

MEAL	TIME	FOOD/ BEVERAGE INTAKE	HOW DO YOU FEEL (tired, bloated, hungry, etc.)
BREAKFAST			
SNACK			
LUNCH			
SNACK			
DINNER			
SNACK			

DAY FIVE

MEAL	TIME	FOOD/ BEVERAGE INTAKE	HOW DO YOU FEEL (tired, bloated, hungry, etc.)
BREAKFAST			
SNACK			
LUNCH			
SNACK			
DINNER			
SNACK			

DAY SIX

MEAL	TIME	FOOD/ BEVERAGE INTAKE	HOW DO YOU FEEL (tired, bloated, hungry, etc.)
BREAKFAST			
SNACK			
LUNCH			
SNACK			
DINNER			
SNACK			

DAY SEVEN

MEAL	TIME	FOOD/ BEVERAGE INTAKE	HOW DO YOU FEEL (tired, bloated, hungry, etc.)
BREAKFAST			
SNACK			
LUNCH			
SNACK			
DINNER			
SNACK			

What the Fork Plan of Action

Did you get lazy and record only three days? Well, have no fear—you still have something to work with. So, let's dig in and assess what you are eating. This is not a test; it's a simple, thought-provoking activity that could very well be your wake-up call. By understanding, on paper, what you eat (and how you do so), the *real* obstacles preventing you from making healthier choices typically shine through, and then solutions are much easier to come by. Let the games begin.

1. What do you generally eat for breakfast?
   - ❑ Nothing
   - ❑ Just coffee or tea
   - ❑ Something processed, such as anything fast food; boxed cereal; pastries and muffins; sugared yogurts

❑ Something more wholesome, such as eggs; fresh fruit; a fresh fruit smoothie; vegetable juice (or a green drink); oatmeal; a less-processed cereal like muesli or a low-sugar granola; plain yogurt

Readiness/willingness to change:

❑ I want/need to change

❑ I don't want to/can't change

2. **What do you generally eat for lunch?**

❑ Nothing

❑ Fast food; other type of takeout (and not necessarily healthy)

❑ Canned soups; lunch meats, whether in sandwiches or salads

❑ Soups; raw or cooked vegetables; whole grains; legumes, fish, poultry, or meat

Readiness/willingness to change:

❑ I want/need to change

❑ I don't want to/can't change

3. **What do you generally eat for dinner?**

❑ Nothing

❑ Fast food; other greasy takeout

❑ Canned soups; lunch meats, whether in sandwiches or salads

❑ Soups; raw or cooked vegetables; whole grains; legumes, fish, poultry, or meat

Readiness/willingness to change:

❑ I want/need to change

❑ I don't want to/can't change

4. **What do you generally eat for snacks?**

❑ Nothing

❑ Diet beverages

❏ Something highly processed with lots of sugar, such as beverages;
   candy; cookies; cakes; pastries; protein bars; super-salty and
   overflavorful chips and crackers

❏ Fresh fruit; vegetables; bean dip; eggs; cheese; yogurt; nuts and seeds;
   minimally processed crackers

Readiness/willingness to change:

❏ I want/need to change

❏ I don't want to/can't change

5. **What do you generally drink throughout the day?**

❏ Sugared beverages

❏ Coffee

❏ Unsweetened beverages such as tea or coconut water

❏ Water or seltzer

Readiness/willingness to change:

❏ I want/need to change

❏ I don't want to/can't change

6. **How many times do you have sweets (other than fresh fruit) during the day?**

❏ 5 or more

❏ 3 to 5

❏ 1 to 3

❏ 0 to 1

Readiness/willingness to change:

❏ I want/need to change

❏ I don't want to/can't change

7. **How many times do you drink alcohol during the week?**

❏ 8 or more

❏ 4 to 8

❑   1 to 4

❑   Never

Readiness/willingness to change:

❑   I want/need to change

❑   I don't want to/can't change

8. Given what you now know about food, how many of your daily choices
    contain the Top-Rated Terminators: chemical preservatives, artificial
    flavors, artificial colors, artificial sweeteners, sugar, and its many
    euphemisms, trans fats, and so on?

    ❑   5 or more

    ❑   3 to 5

    ❑   1 to 3

    ❑   None

    Readiness/willingness to change:

    ❑   I want/need to change

    ❑   I don't want to/can't change

9. How many Can't Live Withouts do you consume in a day?

    ❑   5 or more

    ❑   3 to 5

    ❑   1 to 3

    ❑   0 to 1

    Readiness/willingness to change:

    ❑   I want/need to change

    ❑   I don't want to/can't change

Consider yourself self-assessed. Now what to do with this? How
about trying to set some realistic goals (see sidebar, "How Do You Plan to
Take Action—a Helping Hand" on page 232 for a little insight)?

Name Three Things You Would Like to Change about Your Food Choices

1.

2.

3.

Name Three Obstacles Preventing You from Changing What You Eat

1.

2.

3.

Name Three Things You Can Realistically Change about What You Eat in the
Next Month (Your Goals)

1.

2.

3.

Explain How You Plan to Take Action (see sidebar, "How Do You Plan to Take
Action—A Helping Hand," page 232) and Make the Changes You Named
(How You Plan to Reach Your Goals)

1.

2.

3.

One of the best pieces of advice someone ever gave me was, "Stefanie, the slower you go, the faster you get there." Thus, know that whatever you do now (or later) is a step in the right direction. I will say it again: Small changes can make big everyday differences.

How Do You Plan to Take Action— a Helping Hand

Confused? Here are some ideas for a plan of action, but remember, yours will depend on what goals you are setting, and the following is just a sampling:

1. I will wake up ten minutes earlier so I can eat breakfast every morning.
2. I will have a wholesome breakfast three mornings a week instead of my regular bagel with cream cheese.
3. I will have a salad for lunch three days a week.
4. I will choose foods without the Top-Rated Terminators.
5. I will cook two to three nights a week or more if possible.
6. I will eat regularly throughout the day, aiming not to skip any meals.

What the Fork Food Philosophy

If it were up to me, you'd be eating a 70 to 80 percent whole-foods diet, with lots of variety, composed of a wholesome breakfast, lunch, and dinner with two to three snacks throughout the day. You wouldn't skip meals and you would surely eat at regular intervals. None of your foods would have any of the Top-Rated Terminators and you would get your butt in the kitchen and cook mostly everything yourself. But what planet am I living on? And as I said, the slower you go, the faster you get there.

I am by no means trying to oversimplify the complex process of changing food habits and behaviors, but I can assure you that you finally have a new food toolkit to help you better balance your plate. One more thing before taking a walk with me to the wild side—that is, the kitchen: Here is

	MON	TUES	WED	THURS	FRI	SAT	SUN
BREAKFAST 7–8 A.M. Water, tea, coffee	Wrapped-Up Eggs and Veg (p 245)	Power Green (or other smoothie p. 242)	Oatmeal Cookie Oatmeal (p. 247)	Plain yogurt with Golicious Granola (p. 248)	Berry Smooth (or other smoothie p. 243) / Hard-boiled egg	Tofu Rambling Scramble (p. 246)	Grandma Helen's Pancakes (p. 249)
SNACK 10–11 A.M. Water or other unsweetened beverage	Mixed nuts or nut-and-dried-fruit bar; granola or health-bent "cookie"; fresh fruit; apple with nut butter; fruit and vegetable smoothie; fresh vegetables (or crackers) with dip such as hummus; soup; hard-boiled egg; yogurt; cheese with crackers; dark chocolate square						
LUNCH 12–1 P.M. Water or other unsweetened beverage	Lazy Lentil Soup (p. 268)	Greens and Beans Salad (p. 252)	Untraditional Egg Salad (p. 284) alone, in a wrap or on whole grain bread	Cheesy Bok Choy Caesar Salad (p. 254)	Crunchy Cabbage Slaw (p. 255)	Spiked Cilantro Hummus (p. 279)	Easy Creamy Tomato Dill Soup (p. 267)
	Greek Goddess Salad (p. 251)			Chicken and Rice Soup (p. 266)	Cowgirl Chili (p. 281)	Red Quinoa Tabouli (p. 274)	Dirty Lentils (p. 280)
SNACK 3–4 P.M. Water or other unsweetened beverage	CHOOSE FROM SNACK OPTIONS IN FIRST SNACK SECTION						
DINNER 6–7 P.M. Water or other unsweetened beverage	VEGETABLE Green salad dressed with vinaigrette AND/OR steamed/grilled/baked/sautéed vegetables STARCH ½ cup cooked grain (brown rice, quinoa, polenta, pasta) OR small baked potato OR ½ cup cooked squash OR ½ cup beans PROTEIN 3 to 4 ounces grilled/baked/broiled fish/poultry/meat OR vegetarian option						
SNACK	CHOOSE FROM SNACK OPTIONS IN FIRST SNACK SECTION (if hungry)						

a sample weekly menu (my *very* basic ideal,* calling on some recipes from *What the Fork* assuming you have no food allergies and sensitivities). But do know that it's simply a guide. I don't expect you to get in the kitchen (though if you can, great), to hand-craft every meal. If you can't or don't want to make it, aim to substitute like dishes from other kitchens.

*Note that this menu reflects the foundation of a healthy diet. But it is not intended to offer specific dietary guidance based on individual needs.

CHAPTER 17

Recipe Rehab

A little on my inner cook: Put me in the kitchen and there are no boundaries. And perhaps this has to do with observing my mom. For example, once when I was in high school, after a long day of classes topped off by soccer practice, my brother and I arrived home to a meal of scrambled eggs and toast. This was *breakfast for dinner*. While my brother was beside himself complaining that this couldn't possibly be a real dinner, I thought this was creative genius. My mom was always doing things a little differently and I happily emulated that part of her. I don't follow any set of culinary rules; I cook with what is accessible with variety in mind and shape that around what I'm in the mood for and what I feel my body needs; plus food is balanced based on color, texture, flavor, and, yes—nutrition. That's a mouthful!

When I was being trained at Annemarie Colbin's Natural Gourmet Institute for Health and Culinary Arts, the sole focus was food as health. Each and every ingredient we worked with was pure—meaning not one contained a Top-Rated Terminator. So while I hope that you aim to thoughtfully purchase all ingredients, I am done pestering you. You now have the tools to navigate food and I trust that you will do the best that you can.

My goal with everything edible is to take common culinary delights like granola, Caesar salad, cream of tomato soup, egg salad, chili, meat loaf, and even caramel and put a healthier yet quite tasty spin on these sumptuous selections. All my recipes are pretty simple to make, and they are chock-full of ingredients that aren't too weird and are pretty easy to find. There are options for the plant lover, meat eater, and everything in between, and nutritious meets delicious in every one (except perhaps the caramel recipe). I come from a fairly filterless, highly opinionated family with mainstream palates. If they love a good portion of my food, then I imagine you will as well.

Oh, and another thing: I don't drink, so if you ask me about wine and how to pair with food, you will get a blank stare. But ask me how to pair food with food, and you'll want to shut me up. So to help you balance your plate, I have paired many of the recipes (mostly with other recipes from this book) to make planning wholesome meals easy peasy, and with this and the sample weekly menu, you should have every opportunity to put your best foot forward. Finally, each recipe has a story to tell, so read it and eat.

Not-So-Kitschy Kitchen Equipment

Whether I am working with a private client or teaching a group, this inevitable question comes up: "What is your favorite kitchen gadget?" Folks, let's get something straight—I don't do many gadgets. But my go-to pieces of equipment are my Cuisinart (aka food processor), Vitamix (aka super-extraordinary blender), citrus press, and Microplane (a razor-sharp etched-steel contraption that finely grates everything from ginger to cheese). My most cherished and used tools (because that is another question often asked) are my chef's knife (Global is my brand of preference) and cast-iron pans. So for kitchen equipment, I don't go kitschy. I go basic and I suggest you do the same (by the way, you don't need *everything* on this list):

POTS/PANS (Avoid nonstick)*

❑   4- to 6-quart pot (stainless steel)

❑   8-quart stockpot (stainless steel)

*Steer clear of all nonstick cooking surfaces. Most pans are metal coated with a synthetic substance called polytetrafluoroethylene (PTFE), also known as Teflon (compliments of DuPont). According to tests conducted by the Environmental Working Group, "In just two to five minutes on a conventional stove top, cookware coated with Teflon and other non-stick surfaces could exceed temperatures at which the coating breaks apart and emits toxic particles and gases."[1] In fact, the chemicals released upon heating can kill pet birds and is suspected to cause "Teflon flu" (a fever associated with inhalation of the fumes). Sounds pretty gnarly to me overall. While there are safer nonstick surfaces these days like Scan Pan, I steer clear of anything with a coating or added chemicals.

- ❑ 10- to 12-inch frying pan (stainless steel or cast iron)

- ❑ Large sauté pan (stainless steel or cast iron)

- ❑ Grill pan (stainless steel or cast iron)

- ❑ Wok (stainless steel)

- ❑ Clay pot (Romertopf is a good choice)

OVENWARE (Avoid nonstick)*

- ❑ Baking sheets, with edges

- ❑ Cupcake pans (small and large)

- ❑ Loaf pans (glass or ceramic)

- ❑ Baking dishes (glass or ceramic)

UTENSILS

- ❑ (If you opt for plastic, as they are often less expensive, make sure they are BPA-free)

- ❑ Knives (stainless steel; a chef's knife and paring knife will suffice for the basic cook)

- ❑ Knife sharpener (the sharpener can be as basic as an $8–$10 stone that sharpens your blade just as well as the more fancy and expensive kinds, so don't get fooled; consider sharpening your blade a few times a year)

- ❑ Knife steel (this wandlike rod hones your blade between sharpenings, giving the knife an acute adjustment; it can be used as often as you like)

- ❑ Cutting boards, preferably wooden or bamboo; a good BPA-free plastic board works too (see the following sidebar, "On Cutting Boards, page 238")

- ❑ Wooden spoons (assorted)

- ❑ Large mixing spoon (stainless steel)

- ❑ Slotted spoon (stainless steel)

- ❑ Ladle (stainless steel)

- ❑ Tongs (stainless steel)

- ❑ Spatula (stainless steel)

- ❏ Rubber spatula

- ❏ Whisk

- ❏ Potato masher

- ❏ Peeler

- ❏ Lemon/lime press

- ❏ Grater/shredder/Microplane

- ❏ Can opener

- ❏ Measuring cups (stainless steel and glass)

- ❏ Measuring spoons (stainless steel)

OTHER

- ❏ Mixing bowls (stainless steel and glass)

- ❏ Blender

- ❏ Food processor

- ❏ Glass storage containers

On Cutting Boards

When selecting cutting boards, which way do you go? I am a fan of wood, bamboo, and plastic (BPA-free) and won't touch glass (and suggest that you don't) primarily because I find that my knife slips when cutting and the glass blunts my blade (both utterly unsafe). So here is my take:

WOOD AND BAMBOO

I use both porous boards for plant and animal foods but always make sure that I have a separate board for each (meaning that I have four specific boards—plants, fish, poultry, and meat). Wood and bamboo are kind to my knife (meaning the blade doesn't easily dull) and because both give just a little, cutting is super safe. Food can get stuck in the pores of the wood (and grooves from knives) so a good cleaning is essential (and a little laborious for both materials). To clean I like to give my boards the spa treatment—hot water, soap, lemon (or vinegar) and salt, then a good dry with a clean kitchen towel. And as both wood and bamboo can warp, keeping them oiled after a good cleaning helps the moisture stay in. If your board is crisscrossed with grooves, it's time for a new one. A note on bamboo: This fast-growing *grass* is considered the best choice for the more eco-minded person.

PLASTIC

Plastic cutting boards are often thought to be a better option than porous wood, but think again. Yes, they are incredibly durable and last longer (no oiling required), don't destroy a knife's blade, and are *thought* to clean more easily than wood (a quick wash with hot water and soap or a toss in the dishwasher), but there are some concerns about these polyethylene plastic boards. According to the late Dr. Dean Cliver, a noted scientist, researcher, and professor who extensively studied infectious agents in food and water, bacteria on plastic boards, *especially those that are scarred*, don't die even with hot soapy water or a run through the dishwasher (in fact, bacteria on the boards simply transfer to other surfaces in the dishwasher). While wood harbors bacteria as well, Cliver notes that microbes that propagate will eventually die off.[2] Bottom line, if your plastic is groovy, replace it. Or you can soak it nightly in a bleach solution to kill off *most* of the bacteria (1 tablespoon of bleach to 1 gallon of water), though not my favored way to go.

And while there are other types of cutting boards on the market, such as Epicurean (wood fibers compressed with a food-safe resin) and I encourage you to try others on for size, the most accessible (and cost-effective) for the uncommon cook are wood, bamboo, and plastic. No matter which material you choose to use, be sure to have one for plants and another for meats (perhaps three if you are like me) to prevent cross-contamination.

On Microwaves

Once when teaching a cooking immersion program, I had a husband-wife combo as students—he cooked on the stove and in the oven; she made everything happen in a microwave. They wouldn't have it any other way. But they were curious about two things: (1) Do I use a microwave? and (2) What do I think about this magical "oven"? No, I don't have a microwave, nor do I use one (unless I am somewhere with no other option). Honestly, I just don't trust them. And this is why in a nutshell: *Environmental Nutrition*, a highly credible, consumer-friendly industry newsletter on nutrition, environment, and health has this to offer regarding the safety of these innovative food machines:

> Radiation emissions have been a big concern for consumers. However, the FDA regulates the amount of emissions microwaves can emit over an oven's lifetime, to a level established as safe. As an additional precaution, the FDA requires two systems of backup security and monitoring to shut down the microwave if a system dysfunctions or a door opens while in use. The FDA suggests that consumers stand away from a microwave when it's in use to significantly reduce microwave radiation exposure, and never to operate a microwave if the door or hinges are bent, damaged or improperly sealed.[3]

Why don't I have or use a microwave? You are supposed to stand away from the machine when it is working to limit your exposure to radiation, but it's okay for you to consume zapped food. That just makes no real sense to me. I prefer food cooked traditionally, without too much technology. However, you decide for yourself.

Break the Fast with Breakfast

Breakfast literally means breaking the fasting period of the prior night (while you were sleeping, that is). It is the most important meal of the day, as it sets the tone for how you will eat throughout your waking hours. According to WebMD, skipping meals, especially breakfast, leads to eating more food than usual at the next meal or nibbling on high-calorie snacks to ward off hunger.[4] So don't just dabble in breakfast, do it. Whether you have five minutes or fifteen, there's an option for you.

Power Green
Berry Smooth
Banananutty
Wrapped-Up Eggs and Veg
Tofu Rambling Scramble
Oatmeal Cookie Oatmeal
Golicious Granola
Grandma Helen's Pancakes

Power Green | Berry Smooth | Banananutty

I am not so jazzed about juicing. It can surely complement a healthy food–based diet, but most opt for one of the "fabulous faddist" juice cleanses, and quite honestly, they can be downright dangerous (see the sidebar, "The Juice on Juicing," page 244).

Juicing, in the more traditional fashion—like fresh from your own high-powered juicer or what you would buy in a bottle from one of those hip juice-cleanse companies—rips valuable fiber out of the fruits and vegetables being compressed. Folks, that fiber is good stuff. So my answer to juicing is FUICING—food as "juice." And I use my trusty Vitamix (that super-powered blender like no other) to purée my food into fuice. But a regular blender can do the trick, too.

Each of the three recipes that follow relies on some form of milk (plain rice milk is my preference), fresh frozen fruits, and lots of other goodness. Truth be told, my breakfast almost every day begins with the Power Green. and I drink the whole darn thing, knowing that I am getting nourished in the way my body needs. Not that I am urging each and every one of you to suck down 32 ounces; it is a lot (though you can actually save the extra in the fridge for later in the day). So definitely share among family members or cut the recipe in half. And if you just have a little bit and want some other morning nourishment, pair it with an egg or two (cooked any style), a little yogurt, or some Golicious Granola (page 248). Happy juicing . . .

Power Green   MAKES 32 OZ.

INGREDIENTS:

    1½ cups plain rice milk or other milk (dairy or nondairy)

    ½ cup ice

    1 cup kale leaves, loosely packed (or a large handful)

    ½ cup flat-leaf parsley, loosely packed (or a small handful)

    2-inch piece cucumber (if waxed [skin is super shiny and slippery],
        then peel)

    ½ cored apple, skin on

    ½ avocado

    ½ ripe banana, frozen

    1¼-inch slice fresh ginger root, peeled

    Juice of 1 lime

METHOD:

    Combine all ingredients, liquid first, in a blender and purée until smooth.

STEFANIE'S NOTES

    When freezing bananas, peel them, break them in half, and store them in a bag or container; and feel free to use other herbs such as mint, cilantro, and basil to complement or replace the parsley.

Berry Smooth

INGREDIENTS:

1½ cups plain rice milk or other milk (dairy or nondairy)

1 cup pure coconut water

2 cups frozen berries (no added sugar)

½ avocado

¼ cup raw almonds

1 teaspoon honey or pure maple syrup

METHOD:

Combine all ingredients, liquid first, in a blender and purée until smooth.

STEFANIE'S NOTES

You can also use other nuts like pecans or eliminate the nuts altogether and replace with 2 tablespoons of flax meal; for an easy snack, freeze in ice cube trays or as ice pops for later.

Banananutty

INGREDIENTS:

1½ cups plain rice milk or other milk (dairy or nondairy)

1 cup ice

2 large ripe bananas, frozen

2 tablespoons almond butter

2 tablespoons flax meal

½ teaspoon ground cinnamon

METHOD:

Combine all ingredients, liquid first, in a blender and purée until smooth.

When freezing bananas, peel them, break them in half, and store them in a bag or container; for an easy snack, freeze this recipe in ice cube trays or as ice pops for later.

The Juice on Juicing

A few years ago my dear friend Allison called and said, "You won't believe what I did, and please don't scold me." I could sense a measure of stress in her voice.

Turns out Allison decided to jump on the juice-cleanse "fad wagon" and signed up for one of those hip and trendy New York City cleanses. The problem: Allison is hypoglycemic (has a long history of low blood sugar) and is prone to migraines. Knowing this, she opted to dine on some vegetables along with the juice, but as the first day progressed, so did the migraine, vomiting, and dehydration. Quite a pickle Allison was in.

As this particular cleanse company did not have a 1-800-PLS-HELP hotline with a health professional guiding the ill-fated customer, Allison spoke to a receptionist, who said, "Sorry, we can't help you. Go to the emergency room." So that's when she called me.

It is important to understand that when cleansing, you can experience mild to severe symptoms including decreased energy, headaches, nausea, rashes, altered bowel movements, and miscellaneous discomforts. So this process should *never* be taken lightly.

If Allison's health history had been reviewed by a health professional before she signed up for this cleanse, she could have avoided the inevitable—her blood sugar dropping dramatically (drinking just juice throughout the day—even with a few veggies in between—lends itself to a rapid rise, then fall, in blood sugar, even if the juice is healthy). Anyone with any medical nutrition expertise would never have put my friend on a juice-centric cleanse. In the end, you are responsible for your own health, but often you get sucked into the fad without forethought.

Food is medicine, and if not administered responsibly, it can hurt. And many of these juice cleanses are not administered with the support of credible health professionals; thus I hold these companies responsible on many levels. They are "bottom-line businesses." According to *Environmental Nutrition*, "Juicing is on the fast-track from fad to full-on health craze. But as healthy as these juicy concoctions may seem, there's a tall order of hype muddling science with slick marketing."[5] In fact, despite what you may hear or read, there is no *hard* scientific evidence supporting the health benefits of juice cleansing.

Although the medical community essentially dismisses juice cleansing as a baseless fad and potentially harmful, I believe it has its place if done properly and responsibly. If you are embarking on a juice cleanse, always seek guidance from a credible medical or nutrition professional, and I beg you to reveal your complete medical history (not a stone unturned). Also, make sure to limit, if not stop, physical activity; always ease your way into a cleanse and out of a cleanse (you don't want to go from eating steak and potatoes one day to only juices the next); ideally, go with a food-based cleanse (primarily plant-centric, perhaps a little fish) combined with lots of water, healthy fuices (or juices), and supplements only if deemed necessary by your practitioner.

Wrapped-Up Eggs and Veg   SERVES 1

This is a morning favorite in our house. Whether pan-fried or boiled, the egg is always central, but depending on who is at the helm of the wrap on the morning of its making, ingredients can shift like the wind. Sometimes it's melted cheddar instead of goat cheese, and often that goes hand in hand with a smack of salsa. Any way you slice it, this wrap is seriously scrumptious.

INGREDIENTS:

1 teaspoon extra virgin olive oil

1 large egg

1 tortilla, warmed

1 tablespoon goat cheese

¼ avocado

Crushed red pepper flakes (optional)

½ cup arugula, loosely packed

METHOD:

1. Heat the olive oil in a small pan over medium heat. Add the egg and fry it to your liking.

2. While the egg is cooking, heat the tortilla in a low oven or even on the stovetop in a dry pan, for about 2 minutes. When the tortilla is warm, spread the goat cheese on the tortilla, scoop the avocado from its skin, layer the avocado on top of the cheese, then sprinkle with red pepper flakes (if using). Add the finished egg and top with arugula. Wrap as you would a burrito.

STEFANIE'S NOTES

You can use a flour, corn, or gluten-free tortilla, and don't forget the salsa if you want an extra zing.

Tofu Rambling Scramble   SERVES 4

For the vegan, this is your yellow scramble but eggless. It's delish on a slice of grainy bread or a tortilla or even stuffed in a pita pocket. My preference is mixing it with some warm rice, whether white or brown. And while it's surely suitable for your morning munch, it doesn't discriminate against other meals.

INGREDIENTS:

2 tablespoons extra virgin olive oil

1 medium red bell pepper, small dice

1 small yellow squash, small dice

2 to 3 large scallions, thinly sliced

1½ teaspoons curry powder

½ teaspoon ground cumin

1 block extra-firm tofu, drained and crumbled

2 tablespoons tamari or soy sauce

¼ teaspoon salt, or more to taste

METHOD:

1. In a large sauté pan, heat the olive oil over medium heat. Add the bell pepper, squash, and scallions, then toss and cook for 2 minutes. Add the curry powder and cumin and mix well. Let cook for another 2 minutes.

2. Drain tofu from water, wrap in 3 layers of paper towels, and press gently to remove excess water. Then crumble the tofu by hand (small to medium pieces) into the pan and mix well. Add the tamari and salt, mix well, and cook for another few minutes, tossing regularly.

STEFANIE'S NOTES

Tamari is a type of soy sauce made typically from soybeans with a touch of wheat (and sometimes no wheat at all). Soy sauce, as most know it, is usually made from equal parts soybeans and wheat. Tamari is richer in flavor and pretty easy to come by these days. Store the Rambling Scramble in the fridge for two to three days; it's great cold for lunch and reheats well. Do not freeze, as tofu changes texture when frozen and can become unpalatable.

Oatmeal Cookie Oatmeal   SERVES 1 TO 2

Oatmeal is super simple to make and doesn't have to be boring. So throw away those oversugared packets of highly processed "oatmeal," grab some rolled oats (even some quick oats if you must), and turn this nutritious dish into a delightfully delicious and desserty kind of breakfast. This is one of my kids' winter favorites.

INGREDIENTS:

½ cup rolled oats

¼ cup water

1 cup rice milk or other milk (dairy or nondairy)

½ teaspoon ground cinnamon

⅛ teaspoon ground nutmeg

Maple syrup, to taste

2 tablespoons chopped walnuts (optional)

1 tablespoon currants (optional)

METHOD:

In a small pot, combine the oats, water, milk, cinnamon, and nutmeg and cook over medium heat, mixing occasionally, until the liquid is absorbed and the oats are soft, 5 to 10 minutes. Add maple syrup to taste and top with the walnuts and currants.

Golicious Granola   SERVES 4 TO 6

This granola is my answer to a healthy breakfast, whether it is served plain or with milk or yogurt. It also more than suffices as a snack. And my son Jack loves it atop an evening bowl of ice cream. Why "golicious"? Well, when Jack was little, he couldn't say "delicious."

INGREDIENTS:

½ cup whole raw almonds, coarsely chopped by hand or with a food processor

½ cup pecans, coarsely chopped by hand or with a food processor

½ cup walnuts, coarsely chopped by hand or with a food processor

½ cup rolled oats

¼ cup flax meal

¼ cup unsweetened coconut

¼ teaspoon ground cinnamon

⅛ teaspoon ground cloves

1 teaspoon pure vanilla extract

1 tablespoon honey

¼ cup brown rice syrup

1 tablespoon coconut oil, unmelted

Pinch of salt

METHOD:

1. Preheat the oven to 325°F.

2. Combine all ingredients in a large bowl and mix thoroughly with either a wooden spoon or your clean hands, ensuring that the coconut oil is evenly mixed throughout.

3. Cover a baking sheet with parchment and spread the mixture on the baking sheet in one thin layer; bake for 10 minutes, then mix on the baking sheet and bake for another 10 minutes.

4. Remove from the oven and allow the granola (that may be a little tender) to cool for 15 minutes before breaking it into chunks.

STEFANIE'S NOTES

Many ovens are not calibrated, meaning that food cooks unevenly. This granola can burn easily so keep a close eye on it as you are cooking to prevent burning. Store in an airtight container in a cool, dry place for up to one week. Or store it in the fridge or freezer, as it lasts longer, anywhere from one to three months. As this granola isn't super sweet, there is no shame in drizzling a little honey or maple syrup over your edible bowl.

Grandma Helen's Pancakes   MAKES TWO 8-INCH PANCAKES

My husband's mother, Helen, was Polish, but during World War II she moved to France, where she was raised. She adored cooking and married both countries' culinary delicacies when creating anything edible. My husband now pays it forward and makes these pancakes (half Polish pancake, and half French crêpe) for our boys. To add some powerful nutrition, top with a little plain yogurt, berries, and nuts. And you can't forget the real maple syrup.

INGREDIENTS:

    2 large eggs
    ½ cup milk or other milk (dairy or nondairy)
    ½ teaspoon pure vanilla extract
    ¼ teaspoon ground cinnamon
    ¼ cup flour (whole wheat, spelt, or gluten-free)
    1 tablespoon butter

METHOD:

1. In a medium bowl, combine the eggs, milk, vanilla, and cinnamon. Whisk until blended and slowly add the flour while still mixing.

2. In an 8-inch pan, melt the butter over medium heat. Add half of the batter and cook the pancake for 3 minutes or until you see small bubbles on the top surface of the pancake. Flip and cook for another 1 to 2 minutes. Before making the second pancake, be sure to remix the remaining batter.

3. Serve with fresh fruit and maple syrup.

Very Vegetable

Veggies need love. If fresh and local (even not so local), they are delish in the raw. But any way you chop it, they can use a little flavor. When my son Jack was little, instead of introducing steamed and puréed plants, I added a little zest to dazzle his palate. In my humble opinion, many kids turn a blind eye to their vegetables because their first experience of them is flavorless.

After years in the kitchen and working with people in their kitchens, I am convinced that the most *underutilized* (and most medicinal) edibles are herbs and spices. Why? Because people don't know how to use them, whether alone or combined with other aromatics, and quite honestly, dried herbs and spices are packaged in such large jars that spending the money on these culinary scents seems foolish when they will only be used a couple of times before they expire. So if you learn how to simply slip flavor into your plants, then maybe you'd eat more veggies and your little loved ones would too.

By the way, make sure you wash everything (even if organic). And as mentioned earlier in the book, say sayonara to the sprays and clean your produce with some good old-fashioned water, rubbing with your hands. If you don't want to mess up your mitts, buy a natural-fiber vegetable brush to do your scrubbing. Oh, and salad spinners are the perfect "car wash" for greens, even for the triple washed.

Greek Goddess Salad
Greens and Beans Salad
Cucumber Mint Salad
Cheesy Bok Choy Caesar Salad
Crunchy Cabbage Slaw
Skillet Broccoli
Shards of Brussels with Herbed Dijon
Wilted Greens
Kale Ratatouille
Naked Eggplant Parmesan

Greek Goddess Salad   SERVES 4 TO 6

You just can't beat a good Greek salad. Instead of the common iceberg lettuce, I use romaine to pack this puppy with nutrition. This bowl of greens and things is simple to make and is as gorgeous as a goddess. Toss in some chicken, a can of sardines or some chickpeas, and lunch away.

FOR SALAD:

  1 medium head romaine lettuce, shredded

  1 medium cucumber, cut into half-moons (if waxed, peel)

  1 pint grape tomatoes, halved

  2 large scallions, thinly sliced

  ¼ cup pitted Kalamata olives

  ½ pound feta cheese, small dice (or crumbled)

  ½ cup mint leaves, loosely packed, roughly chopped

FOR DRESSING:

  2 tablespoons extra virgin olive oil

  ¼ cup fresh lemon juice

  ¼ teaspoon salt

METHOD:

  Combine all of the salad ingredients in a medium bowl. In a small bowl, combine the dressing ingredients and mix well; add to the salad ingredients and toss.

PAIR WITH:

  Lazy Lentil Soup (page 268)
  Cornmeal-Crusted Chicken Cutlets (page 292)

Greens and Beans Salad   SERVES 4

This salad is a cinch—lunch 1-2-3. While it is ideal to cook your own beans, who has the time? Let me ease your pain by telling you that eating canned beans is just fine if it means that you will eat them. If you don't like white beans, use whatever nugget you fancy to make this salad complete.

INGREDIENTS:

1 15-ounce can white beans (cannellini), drained and rinsed

1 cup cherry or grape tomatoes, halved

½ avocado, medium dice

1 small shallot, minced

2 tablespoons chopped fresh dill

1 tablespoon extra virgin olive oil

¼ cup fresh lime juice

¼ teaspoon salt

Freshly ground black pepper, to taste

4 cups arugula, loosely packed

METHOD:

1. Drain and the rinse beans in a fine-mesh strainer; place them in a medium salad bowl and combine with the tomatoes, avocado, shallot, dill, olive oil, lime juice, and salt. Mix well and season with pepper to taste.

2. Serve on a bed of arugula.

STEFANIE'S NOTES

The bean salad can go solo (without the arugula) and can last for two to three days in the fridge. Great for lunch or even a snack.

PAIR WITH:

Skillet Broccoli (page 256)

Savory Herb-Roasted Chicken (page 294)

Cucumber Mint Salad   SERVES 4 TO 6

This quick and cooling salad is perfect to soften the spice of any dish. Eaten right away, it crunches in your mouth with fireworks of flavor. If saved for the day after, the cukes are officially pickled, mildly soft, and even better.

INGREDIENTS:

   2 large, unpeeled seedless cucumbers, cut into ¼-inch rounds

   2 tablespoons red onion, small dice

   ¼ cup mint leaves, loosely packed, roughly chopped

   2 tablespoons extra virgin olive oil

   ¼ cup fresh lemon juice

   ½ teaspoon salt

   Freshly ground black pepper, to taste

METHOD:

   Combine all ingredients in a medium bowl and toss.

PAIR WITH:

   Steamed brown rice (cook as per directions on package)
   Cowgirl Chili (page 281)

Cheesy Bok Choy Caesar Salad   SERVES 4 TO 6

Bok choy is a mystery to many. While most people cook this green, I prefer it raw. Its crunch is followed by a sweet yet slightly edgy flavor, and if it is married with the right dressing, nutritious surely meets delicious here. So this is my take on the more traditional (and somewhat boring) Caesar salad.

FOR SALAD:

   1 head bok choy, roughly chopped

   1 tablespoon red onion, small dice

FOR DRESSING:

   ¼ cup extra virgin olive oil

   1 tablespoon fresh lemon juice

   1 teaspoon Dijon mustard

½ teaspoon black pepper

½ cup shredded Parmesan cheese

METHOD:

1. Combine the bok choy and onion in a large bowl and toss.

2. Combine the olive oil, lemon juice, mustard, pepper, and ¼ cup of the Parmesan and mix until combined either by hand or with a blender. The dressing will still be a little chunky.

3. Toss the dressing with the salad and garnish with the remaining ¼ cup of the Parmesan.

STEFANIE'S NOTES

If you can't find bok choy, use romaine lettuce.

PAIR WITH:

Cooked pasta

Mon Frères Turkey Meatballs (page 295)

Crunchy Cabbage Slaw   SERVES 4 TO 6

My dad loves coleslaw. Watching him consume that pale, often sugared and overcreamy rubbish for years inspired me to find a new way to make this traditional favorite—and one that he would actually eat. While this dish looks different and definitely tastes different from the slaw he is accustomed to, it satisfies his absolutely ordinary palate. So for those who love the mayo, take a bite out of this crunch. You may be surprised.

FOR SALAD:

1 small head purple cabbage, cored, trimmed, and shredded

1 cup leafy green kale, stems removed, loosely packed and shredded

1 large carrot, julienned

FOR DRESSING:

¼ cup extra virgin olive oil

¼ cup rice vinegar

1 tablespoon Dijon mustard

3 tablespoons minced shallot

1 tablespoon chopped fresh thyme leaves

¼ teaspoon salt

METHOD:

1. Combine the cabbage (shredded either by hand or in a food processor), kale, and carrot in a large bowl.

2. In a glass measuring cup or small bowl, whisk the dressing ingredients together.

3. Toss the dressing with the slaw.

STEFANIE'S NOTES

Slaw tastes just as good or even better the day after. So store it in the fridge for your "leftover lunch" for one to two days.

PAIR WITH:

Acorn Squash Chips (page 272)

Fish Tacos (page 285)

Skillet Broccoli   SERVES 4

After years of teaching individuals and groups, it never ceases to amaze me that most people cook broccoli only one way—steamed. Well, folks, if you can relate, how about a twist that can rock your broccoli boat and get pretty much any cruciferous skeptic changing their tune? By the way, most kids prefer their broccoli with a little bang.

INGREDIENTS:

2 tablespoons extra virgin olive oil

1 head broccoli, broken into florets and thinly sliced

Salt, to taste

Freshly ground black pepper, to taste

Juice of ½ lemon (optional)

METHOD:

In a large skillet, heat the olive oil over medium heat. Add the broccoli and let it brown for 2 to 3 minutes, then toss and cook for another 2 to 3 minutes. Finish with salt and pepper; add lemon juice (if using).

STEFANIE'S NOTES

If you don't fancy the skillet, you can always roast this recipe in a 350°F oven for 15 minutes.

PAIR WITH:

Vegetable Fried Rice (page 277)

Teriyaki Salmon (page 288)

Shards of Brussels with Herbed Dijon   SERVES 4

Brussels sprouts can be a bitch. While they are incredibly nutritious, I find few people who actually like them. Roasted whole or halved is the norm, and even then, they are likely unpalatable for many. Determined to get my clients and students to consume them, I tried shredding them (a tad labor intensive) and dazzling them with some dressing after roasting. And lo and behold, now there are many more Brussels believers.

FOR BRUSSELS:

2 pounds Brussels sprouts, bottoms trimmed, halved and thinly sliced

4 tablespoons extra virgin olive oil

¼ teaspoon salt

FOR HERBED DIJON:

½ tablespoon Dijon mustard

3 tablespoons extra virgin olive oil

2 tablespoons brown rice vinegar

1 tablespoon mirin

1 tablespoon minced fresh thyme leaves

1 tablespoon minced fresh oregano leaves

METHOD:

1. Preheat the oven to 350°F.

2. Place the Brussels sprouts in a roasting pan with the olive oil and salt. Toss and spread the sprouts evenly across the pan.

3. Bake for 25 to 30 minutes, turning occasionally, until tender and slightly browned (even a little crispy).

4. Prepare the herbed Dijon by adding ingredients to a bowl and whisking, then toss with the cooked Brussels sprouts.

PAIR WITH:

Curried Sweet Potato Mash (page 270)

Montauk Meat Loaf (page 299)

Wilted Greens   SERVES 4

Greens are good for you. So my job is to help you figure out a way to get these undersonsumed powerhouses into your every day (or almost every day). You can use pretty much any dark leafy green for this recipe. And if it's a little too bitter, cut with something sweet like apple juice—this makes them go down easier for the kids and even many grown-ups.

INGREDIENTS:

2 tablespoons extra virgin olive oil

3 garlic cloves, minced

1 bunch leafy green kale, stems removed, roughly chopped

4 cups baby spinach (or 5-ounce package)

¼ cup water or apple juice

1 teaspoon fresh lemon juice

¼ teaspoon crushed red pepper flakes (optional)

Salt, to taste

METHOD:

1. In a large sauté pan, heat the olive oil over medium heat. Add the garlic and cook for 30 seconds.

2. Add the kale and cook until slightly wilted. Then add the spinach and water or apple juice. Cook for another 2 minutes until the greens are soft. Add the lemon juice, red pepper flakes (if using), and salt.

STEFANIE'S NOTES

Leftover greens are golden. I often finely chop them and add to some eggs while scrambling. Wanna make green eggs for your kids? This surely beats the food dye.

PAIR WITH:

Steamed basmati rice (cook as per directions on package)

Asian Marinated Flank Steak (page 297)

Kale Ratatouille   SERVES 4 TO 6

Once again, a traditional dish with a twist. One of my favorites with pasta or a bowl of rice or just flying solo with a sprinkle of Parmesan. Often I toss this together and throw it on top of a piece of fish for a good old bake in the oven

(350°F for 15 to 20 minutes). Very versatile, highly nutritious, and utterly delicious.

INGREDIENTS:

  2 tablespoons extra virgin olive oil

  2 garlic cloves, minced

  1 medium yellow onion, thinly sliced

  ½ teaspoon dried oregano

  1 teaspoon salt

  1 pint grape tomatoes, left whole

  1 red bell pepper, seeded and thinly sliced

  1 small zucchini, cut into ¼-inch-thick half-moons

  1 large sprig fresh rosemary, or 1 tablespoon dried

  2 large sprigs fresh thyme, or 1 tablespoon dried

  1 medium bunch kale, shredded with stems (about 4 cups packed)

  ½ cup flat-leaf parsley, loosely packed, roughly chopped

METHOD:

  1. In a medium pot, heat the olive oil over medium heat. Add the garlic and onion and sauté for 2 to 3 minutes. Add the oregano, salt, tomatoes, bell pepper, zucchini, rosemary, and thyme. Mix well, cover the pot, and cook on low heat for 30 minutes.

  2. Remove the herb sprigs from the pot and discard. Add the kale and parsley, gently mix, and cook covered for another 3 to 5 minutes.

STEFANIE'S NOTES

  If using dried rosemary and thyme, add them to the pot at the same time as the oregano. This dish is still super delish two to three days after you make it. It can be stored in the freezer for up to three months.

PAIR WITH:

  Steamed quinoa (cook as per directions on package)

  Dirty Lentils (page 280)

Naked Eggplant Parmesan   SERVES 4 TO 6

My grandmother is in her nineties, and her caregiver and dear friend is a woman named Jackie, whom I have grown to love deeply in the twenty-plus years since my grandfather passed away. Jackie is an outstanding cook and loves to nurture me with her culinary creations. One of my favorites is eggplant Parmesan, and this is my take on her recipe. Why naked? 'Cause it's not dressed with egg or bread crumbs.

FOR EGGPLANT:

    2 large eggplants, skin on, sliced ¼ inch thick

    1 28-ounce can crushed tomatoes

    ½ pound hard goat cheese, shredded (or shredded mozzarella)

    ½ cup grated Parmesan cheese

FOR RUB:

    ½ cup extra virgin olive oil

    2 garlic cloves, minced

    2 tablespoons dried oregano

    1 teaspoon salt

METHOD:

1. Preheat the oven to 350°F.

2. Single layer the eggplant slices on two baking sheets. In a small bowl, combine the rub ingredients and mix well. With a fiber brush or rubber spatula, lightly coat both sides of the eggplant with the rub mixture. Bake for 20 minutes.

3. In the bottom of a large baking dish (preferably 4 inches deep), spread ¼ cup of the crushed tomatoes, then layer the eggplant to cover the tomatoes. Top with ½ cup of the tomatoes, then ¼ cup of the cheese (goat and parmesan combined). Repeat layers until done.

4. Cover the baking dish with foil and place it in the oven for 30 minutes.

5. Remove the foil, turn the oven to broil, return the baking dish to the oven, and broil for 5 minutes.

STEFANIE'S NOTES

Although "naked," this dish is quite heavy. You may want to eat it with greens alone and hold the pasta. You can store it in the fridge for two to three days—it can be a yummy lunch or dinner during the week. Store it in the freezer for up to three months.

PAIR WITH:

Wilted Greens (page 258)
Pesto Pasta (page 273)

Seriously Soupy

My mom taught me how to make soups. She is an avid gardener (unlike me) and an artist. So slam the two together and some serious soup is born— colorful, filled with texture, and laced with taste. Growing up, my brother and father were always a tad wary about her "witches' brew," but I always knew that whatever it was, I would feel nourished. My mom encouraged creativity—there were no boundaries—and I seem to have followed in her footsteps with food. Thanks, Mom!

Soups are literally my melting pot of texture, color, flavor, and notorious nutrition. Consider them warming, nurturing, and nourishing. If made with a fine combination of carbohydrates, protein, and fat, a soup can be a brilliant balance of nourishment. These one-pot wonders can make mealtime a breeze too. Make a big pot and put some aside for freezing. They keep well and can feed your soul for months. Don't be shy and soup it up. Every recipe of liquid love is paired, but surely feel free to suck these down solo or with a side salad and a choice chunk of grainy bread.

Must-Have Miso Soup
Cauliflower Cheese Soup
Chicken and Rice Soup
Easy Creamy Tomato Dill Soup
Lazy Lentil Soup

Must-Have Miso Soup

SERVES 4 TO 6

If there is one recipe in this book that boasts weird ingredients, this is it. But I urge you to check the international section at your local market and find what you need to make this easy, nourishing soup. My kids adore it, especially when loaded with some steamed sushi rice. It's the perfect snack, start to a meal, or meal itself when married with a grain. And my boys even eat it for breakfast.

INGREDIENTS:

6 cups water
½ pound tofu, small dice
2 tablespoons wakame seaweed, pre-cut or cut into half-inch pieces
    with scissors
6 tablespoons white miso (not sweet)
¼ cup scallions, thinly sliced
2 teaspoons tamari or soy sauce

METHOD:

1. In a small pot, combine the water, tofu, and wakame and simmer for 10 minutes.

2. Place the miso in a small bowl and add 1½ cups of hot liquid from the pot. Mix until the miso is dissolved, then add it back into the pot.

3. Cook on low for 10 minutes, making sure not to bring the soup to a boil. Garnish with the scallions and tamari.

Miso is whole fermented soybean paste. It boasts beneficial bacteria for your gut (much like anything fermented), so make sure not to boil it when cooking or reheating, as high heat will destroy the bacteria. This soup can be stored in the fridge for up to three days. But do not freeze it, as tofu will change consistency and be quite unpalatable.

PAIR WITH:

Cucumber Mint Salad (page 253)
Asian Marinated Flank Steak (page 298)

Cauliflower Cheese Soup

SERVES 4 TO 6

Cauliflower is a nutrient-dense powerhouse, but unfortunately it is unfavorable to many. So, to get my kids, clients, and students to embrace this cruciferous cupid, cheesing it up was the solution. Lose the cheese if it's not your thing—plain old cauliflower puréed to silkiness is simply delish with a touch of salt and freshly ground black pepper.

INGREDIENTS:

1 large head cauliflower, cut into chunks
4 cups water
1 small yellow onion, thinly sliced
2 cups shredded cheddar cheese
½ teaspoon salt, plus more to taste
Freshly ground black pepper, to taste

METHOD:

1. In a medium pot, combine the cauliflower, water, and onion and cook, covered, over medium heat until the cauliflower is tender, 20 to 30 minutes.

2. Let the soup cool, then place it in a blender with the cheese and ½ teaspoon salt and purée until smooth and creamy. Add more salt and pepper to taste.

STEFANIE'S NOTES

Puréeing warm soups can be a slight kitchen hazard. Take it from me. When puréeing anything hot, to avoid a food explosion, I place a clean dish towel between the top of the blender and its lid, pressing the top down hard with my hands as I let the motor rip. For some scientific reason, this keeps the soup safely in the blender. Feel free to try this technique with any other vegetable—who doesn't love a silky soup? Store in the fridge for up to three days or freeze for up to three months.

PAIR WITH:

Greens and Beans Salad (page 252)
Cornmeal-Crusted Chicken Cutlets (page 292)

A Mean Clean of Anything Animal

Among the many things I learned in culinary school, this was *not* one of them. When cooking at my dear friend's house one evening, unbeknownst to me, I had a sous chef—her Filipina babysitter. All ready to create a fish dish, I pulled the side of salmon out of the fridge to plop in the baking dish when my newly acquired culinary partner grabbed the flesh from my hands and said, "Let me clean that." Stepping aside, I watched this little lady massage the fish with salt and lemon juice, then rinse it under water and pat it dry with a paper towel.

"Stefanie, in my country we always clean flesh, and you should too. Water alone doesn't disinfect like lemon and salt." Often the greatest things we learn don't come from schooling, but life experiences, and I am honored to have learned a thing or two from my unexpected sous chef.

So, as you will note in every recipe containing flesh, whether fish or unground poultry and meat, I ask that you give it a good clean.

Chicken and Rice Soup

SERVES 4 TO 6

My son Jack once said, "Mom, you know those commercials that show kids eating canned soup and they act like it tastes really good? Well, they don't know what good is." Leave it to an eight-year-old! I call this chicken soup for the soul—my boys can literally down a bowl for breakfast, lunch, and dinner. It nourishes in wellness and sickness. Let this soup help take care of you.

INGREDIENTS:

  1 tablespoon extra virgin olive oil

  2 garlic cloves, minced

  1 yellow onion, thinly sliced

  2 carrots, peeled and cut into ¼-inch-thick half-moons

  1 celery stalk, cut into ¼-inch-thick half-moons

  1 chicken breast, skin on, bone in, split

  Juice of ½ lemon, for cleaning chicken

  1 teaspoon salt, for cleaning chicken, plus additional, to taste

  6 cups water

  2 vegetable bouillon cubes (without MSG) (optional)

  ½ bunch flat-leaf parsley, tied with string

  ½ cup brown or white rice

METHOD:

  1. In a large pot, heat the olive oil over medium heat. Add the garlic, onion, carrots, and celery and sauté, occasionally tossing, for 3 minutes until lightly browned.

  2. Clean the chicken with the lemon juice and salt, rinse it under cold water, and pat it dry with a paper towel. Add the chicken to the pot and let it brown for 3 minutes on each side.

3. Add 6 cups of water and the bouillon cubes, parsley, and rice to the pot. Simmer, covered, for 35 minutes or until the internal temperature on the chicken breast reaches 165 degrees.

4. While on simmer, remove the parsley and discard it. Then remove the chicken and shred it into bite-size pieces (discarding the skin and bones). Return the shredded chicken to the pot. Add salt to taste.

STEFANIE'S NOTES

If you are under the weather, add a generous slice of ginger to your soup (discard it when done) and you will have a culinary pharmacy in your pot. Store in the fridge for up to three days or freeze for up to three months.

PAIR WITH:

Cheesy Bok Choy Caesar Salad (page 254)
or
Skillet Broccoli (page 256)
Dirty Lentils (page 280)

Easy Creamy Tomato Dill Soup   SERVES 4 TO 6

Losing the heavy cream for this cream of tomato soup makes it a healthier option than its more conventional counterpart. While using fresh tomatoes would be ideal, unless you live in tomato land or can find some late-summer or early fall selections, the truth is that your fresh red will most likely be tasteless. So cuddle up to some cans of hearty tomato goodness—it's super easy to make and still utterly nutritious and delicious.

INGREDIENTS:

2 tablespoons extra virgin olive oil
2 garlic cloves, thinly sliced
1 small yellow onion, thinly sliced
1 large zucchini, cut into ¼-inch rounds

¼ teaspoon celery seed

¼ teaspoon paprika

1 teaspoon salt

1 28-ounce can crushed tomatoes

1 28-ounce can whole peeled tomatoes

2 tablespoons roughly chopped fresh dill

1 cup grated Parmesan cheese

METHOD:

1. In a large pot, heat the olive oil over medium heat. Add the garlic, onion, zucchini, celery seed, paprika, and salt. Cook for 10 minutes, tossing occasionally.

2. Add the tomatoes, dill, and Parmesan and mix well. Continue cooking, uncovered, for another 20 minutes.

3. Let the soup cool, then place it in a blender and purée until creamy.

PAIR WITH:

Crunchy Cabbage Slaw (page 255)

Zucchini Latkes (page 271)

Baked Buffalo Wings with Creamy Ranch (page 291)

STEFANIE'S NOTES

Be sure to call on my puréeing technique for this soup too. While delish as a soup, it can double as a tomato sauce. Store in the fridge for up to three days or freeze for up to three months.

Lazy Lentil Soup   SERVES 4 TO 6

Of all the beans, lentils are the easiest and quickest to cook. The reds are the laziest—meaning you really don't have to do much to them for a great-tasting dish. And they are packed with protein and other cherished nourishment. If you are feeling a little slothful, give this soup a shot.

INGREDIENTS:

1 tablespoon extra virgin olive oil

2 shallots, thinly sliced

2 celery stalks, thinly sliced

1 cup grape tomatoes, halved

1 sprig fresh rosemary, stem removed, minced

1 cup red lentils

6 cups water

½ teaspoon salt, or more to taste

Freshly ground black pepper, to taste

METHOD:

1. In a medium pot, heat the olive oil over medium heat. Add the shallots, celery, tomatoes, and rosemary and sauté for 3 to 5 minutes or until the vegetables are slightly tender.

2. Add the lentils, water, and ½ teaspoon salt. Bring to a boil, uncovered, over medium heat, then reduce to a simmer and cook for another 30 minutes. Add salt and pepper to taste.

STEFANIE'S NOTES

Store in the fridge for up to three days or freeze for up to three months.

PAIR WITH:

Shards of Brussels with Herbed Dijon (page 257)
Vegetable-Smothered Halibut (page 287)

Somewhat Starchy

Folks, carbohydrates are *not* bad. Most people are hell-bent on believing that super-starchy foods like grains and potatoes (and food products made with both) are harmful to your health. Well, think again. Carbohydrates (that is, anything plant-based, whether veggies, fruit, grains, beans, nuts, or seeds) are an essential part of food selection. You see, they break down into glucose, and that super-cute single sugar molecule is the essence of energy for every body function. So don't go cutting out the carbs; just pick and choose wisely, aiming for the ones that are the least refined—as in the recipes that follow.

Curried Sweet Potato Mash
Zucchini Latkes
Acorn Squash Chips
Pesto Pasta
Red Quinoa Tabouli
Butternut Squash Risotto
Vegetable Fried Rice

Curried Sweet Potato Mash   SERVES 4 TO 6

The good old mashed potato. Toss in some heavy cream, butter, salt, and pepper and you have the heart-attack special on a silver platter. While I must say that I adore the white potato, the sweet boasts far better nutrition, especially when anti-inflammatory curry takes center stage. So try this mash, as it adds a splash of color and culinary creativity to the more pedestrian potato.

INGREDIENTS:

2 large sweet potatoes, skin on, large dice

2 cups water

3 tablespoons extra virgin olive oil

1 small garlic clove, minced

½ teaspoon curry powder

½ teaspoon salt or to taste

½ cup cilantro leaves, loosely packed, roughly chopped

METHOD:

1. In a small pot, combine the sweet potatoes and water. Cover the pot and bring to a boil over medium heat. Reduce to a simmer and cook, covered, until potatoes are soft, 15 to 20 minutes.

2. Using a strainer, drain the water from the potatoes, then return them to the pot (heat off or on simmer) and mash them with a potato masher or fork. Add the remaining ingredients and mix well.

STEFANIE'S NOTES

Store in the fridge for up to three days or freeze for up to three months. When reheating, add a little water to the pot.

PAIR WITH:

Kale Ratatouille (page 259)
Savory Herb-Roasted Chicken (page 294)

Zucchini Latkes   SERVES 4 TO 6 (12 3-INCH PANCAKES)

Growing up Jewish, you learn to love the latke at an early age. My paternal grandmother made them from a box (ugh). Regardless, I remember relishing them every Chanukah. There is just something about food (no matter how good or bad it is) and cultural traditions. This is my less starchy, incredibly homemade version of the potato pancake.

INGREDIENTS:

2 medium unpeeled zucchini, ends trimmed, shredded with a hand
    grater or food processor
1 large unpeeled Idaho potato, shredded with a hand grater or food
    processor
½ small yellow onion, small dice
2 large garlic cloves, minced
2 tablespoons finely chopped parsley

1 large egg

3 tablespoons chickpea or other flour (like wheat, spelt, oat, or rice)

½ teaspoon salt, plus more to taste

½ teaspoon black pepper

¾ cup grapeseed oil or other vegetable oil, for frying

METHOD:

1. Combine the zucchini, potato, onion, garlic, parlsey, egg, flour, ½ teaspoon salt, and pepper in a large bowl. Mix well with a wooden spoon or clean hands.

2. Place the grapeseed oil in a medium sauté pan and preheat over medium-high heat for 5–7 minutes. With a large slotted spoon or spatula, form ¼-inch-thick pancakes, pressing out excess liquid with hands, and ease them into the pan one at a time. Cook for 3 full minutes per side, or until medium brown and crispy. Remove from the oil and set on 3 layers of paper towels to drain. Repeat until done. Salt to taste if needed.

STEFANIE'S NOTES

To make the perfect zucchini latke, your oil needs be hot and the liquid from the latke mixture successfully drained. Store in the fridge for up to three days or freeze for up to three months. Reheat in a 350°F oven. If the latkes are frozen, you may want to wrap them in some foil before placing them in the oven.

PAIR WITH:

Cauliflower Cheese Soup (page 264)

Vegetable-Smothered Halibut (page 287)

Acorn Squash Chips   SERVES 4

Because I am a true lover of the chip, finding ways to create something a tad more nutritious than the plain potato crunch is a quest. Kind of like a sweet potato chip yet not as sweet and not as crunchy, this orange-yellow yum is great as a snack or side to any meal.

INGREDIENTS:

1 large acorn squash, halved and seeded, cut into ¼-inch-thick half-
moons
2 tablespoons extra virgin olive oil
1 teaspoon salt

METHOD:

1. Preheat the oven to 350°F.
2. Spread the squash slices on two baking sheets covered in parchment, and toss with the olive oil and salt. Arrange the slices in a single layer on the baking sheets and bake for 1 hour for a perfectly tender yet crispy chip.

PAIR WITH:

Cucumber Mint Salad (page 253)
Cowgirl Chili (page 281)

Pesto Pasta

SERVES 4 TO 6

Pesto is typically made with cheese. But believe it or not, you can achieve a similar cheesy flavor sans dairy with miso. I created this recipe years ago for a client who needed to stay away from the moo but loved pesto. And it has since stuck. Toss it on pasta or rice; definitely dip your meats in it for some serious flavor before cooking; use it as a great dip for crudités; spread a dollop on some crackers.

INGREDIENTS:

1 12-ounce package dried (or fresh) pasta
8 cups fresh basil leaves, loosely packed
½ cup pine nuts
1 garlic clove

1½ tablespoons white miso (not sweet)

6 tablespoons extra virgin olive oil

½ teaspoon salt, or more to taste

METHOD:

1. Cook the pasta according to the directions on the package.

2. Combine the basil, pine nuts, garlic, miso, olive oil, and salt in a food processor and purée until creamy.

3. When the pasta is done, drain it, place it in a large bowl, and mix with the pesto while still warm.

STEFANIE'S NOTES

If you want the cheese factor, replace the miso with ½ cup grated Parmesan. Store in the fridge for five to seven days or freeze for three to six months. To freeze, plop into ice cube trays or a small storage container. This is the best way to portion pesto for storage.

PAIR WITH:

Greek Goddess Salad (page 251)

Mon Frères Turkey Meatballs (page 295)

Red Quinoa Tabouli

SERVES 4 TO 6

Quinoa contains more protein than any other grainy goodness. So for carb-conscious citizens, this should fall well within your "zone." I am a lover of Middle Eastern eats; thus I have taken this traditional dish (typically made with bulgur wheat) and positioned it with more powerful nutrition. Enjoy the delicate crunch lavished with lemon and lots of flavor in between.

FOR TABOULI:

1 cup red quinoa (or any quinoa)

1½ cups water

½ pint grape tomatoes, quartered

½ seedless cucumber, small dice

2 large scallions, thinly sliced

2 cups flat-leaf parsley, stems removed, loosely packed, roughly chopped

2 garlic cloves, minced

FOR DRESSING:

¼ cup extra virgin olive oil

¼ cup fresh lemon juice

½ teaspoon salt

METHOD:

1. Combine the quinoa and water in a medium pot. Cover and bring to a boil over medium heat; reduce to a simmer and cook until the water is absorbed and the grain is fluffy, 8 to 10 minutes.

2. Combine the tomatoes, cucumber, scallions, parsley, and garlic in a large bowl. When the quinoa is finished, add it to the vegetable mixture and toss. Finish by adding the dressing ingredients directly to the same bowl and mixing well.

STEFANIE'S NOTES

Store in the fridge for up to three days.

PAIR WITH:

Spiked Cilantro Hummus (page 279)

or

Untraditional Egg Salad (page 284)

Butternut Squash Risotto

SERVES 4 TO 6

Who doesn't love risotto? The only concern for me is that it's super heavy given the fact that it is typically made with cream and tons of cheese. I was determined

*to create a lighter option, so consider this a rebirth of a distinct and flavorful
dish. While you may presume that risotto is super labor intensive, think again.
And if you don't fancy butternut squash, try this recipe with any other vegetable
from asparagus to zucchini and anything in between.*

INGREDIENTS:

  2 tablespoons extra virgin olive oil

  1 garlic clove, minced

  1 small yellow onion, small dice

  1 very small butternut squash, peeled and seeded, small dice

  2 small sprigs fresh rosemary, stems removed, minced

  2 cups arborio rice

  6 cups vegetable or chicken broth (you can also use water for lighter
      flavor)

  1 cup grated Parmesan cheese (optional)

  1 teaspoon salt, or more to taste

  Freshly ground black pepper, to taste

METHOD:

  1. In a medium pot, heat the olive oil over medium heat and add the
garlic, onion, squash, and rosemary and sauté for 5 minutes, stirring regularly. Then add the rice and mix well.

  2. Start by pouring 2 cups of the broth into the pot, stirring frequently
until the liquid is absorbed. Repeat with another 2 cups of broth, then a
final 2 cups (the entire process should take about 20 minutes). Turn off the
heat, add the Parmesan (if using), and gently mix. Finish with salt and
pepper.

STEFANIE'S NOTES

  Store in the fridge for up to three days or freeze for up to three months.
When reheating, add a little liquid to the pot.

PAIR WITH:

Greek Goddess Salad (page 251)

or

Wilted Greens (page 258)

Montauk Meat Loaf (page 299)

Vegetable Fried Rice

SERVES 4 TO 6

My take on the more traditional and not-so-healthy Chinese fried rice, this is a family favorite and incredibly versatile. If you don't like brown rice, opt for white. No biggie. And feel free to switch up your veggies or even add some chicken or shrimp for a one-pot powerhouse meal.

INGREDIENTS:

1 cup short-grain brown rice

2 cups water

1 tablespoon sesame oil
    (light in color, similar to any vegetable oil)

1 medium zucchini, small dice

1 small yellow squash, small dice

2 large scallions, thinly sliced

2 tablespoons tamari or soy sauce

2 tablespoons plus 1 teaspoon mirin

1 teaspoon toasted sesame oil (dark brown in color)

METHOD:

1. Place the rice and water in a small pot. Cover and bring to a boil over high heat, then reduce to a simmer and cook for 30 minutes.

2. In a large sauté pan, heat the sesame oil over medium heat. Add the zucchini, squash, and scallions and cook, tossing occasionally, until the vegetables are soft and colors are vibrant, about 5 minutes.

3. Add the finished rice, tamari, and mirin to the pan, mix well, and sauté for another 3 minutes, tossing regularly. Turn off the heat, and toss with the toasted sesame oil.

STEFANIE'S NOTES

On sesame oil, the lighter version is for cooking and the darker, more robust flavored sort is used more as a condiment and ideally should not be heated. Store in the fridge for up to three days or freeze for up to three months. When reheating, add a little liquid to the pot.

PAIR WITH:

Crunchy Cabbage Slaw (page 255)
Asian-Marinated Flank Steak (page 297)

Powerful Proteins

When selecting proteins, aiming to get the aminos from the real deal versus the highly processed junk is your best option. In other words, ditch the fake meats like that phony baloney stuff, the lunch meats, the protein-packed processed foods ranging from cereals, bars, and shakes to chips, cookies, and chocolate; start loving the plant and flesh powerhouses that will pack you with the vital protein you need to keep your structure strong.

Spiked Cilantro Hummus
Dirty Lentils
Cowgirl Chili
Thaied-Up Tempeh
Untraditional Egg Salad
Fish Tacos
Vegetable-Smothered Halibut
Teriyaki Salmon

Macadamia Monkfish
Baked Buffalo Wings with Creamy Ranch
Cornmeal-Crusted Chicken Cutlets
Savory Herb-Roasted Chicken
Mon Frères Turkey Meatballs
Asian Marinated Flank Steak
Montauk Meat Loaf

Spiked Cilantro Hummus   SERVES 4

The late Edith (Deet) Wright was my first culinary mentor. In my late teens, I spent my summer days in the kitchen of Naturally Good in Montauk, New York (then owned by Kathryn Nadeau), cooking alongside this tiny yet incredible tour de force. Deet taught me many things about work ethic, cooking under pressure, and turning out terrific cuisine despite the many challenges facing any cook in a small and insanely busy kitchen. She also taught me how to make a mean hummus—one of my favorites for a snack or light meal. But of course I have wrenched the recipe millions of ways since. And I encourage you to do the same. . . .

INGREDIENTS:

1 15-ounce can garbanzo beans, drained and rinsed
4 tablespoons fresh lemon juice
⅓ cup extra virgin olive oil
1 small garlic clove
¼ cup cilantro leaves, loosely packed
⅛ teaspoon cayenne pepper
½ teaspoon salt or more to taste

METHOD:

Combine all ingredients in a food processor and purée until smooth and creamy. If needed, add more salt to taste.

STEFANIE'S NOTES

If you don't like garbanzos, try this recipe with white beans or even black beans. Store in the fridge for three to five days.

PAIR WITH:

Cucumber Mint Salad (page 253)

or

Red Quinoa Tabouli (page 274)

Dirty Lentils   SERVES 4

Again one of the easiest beans to make, incredibly adaptable, and packed with flavor, lentils just need a little lift to impress the palate. This is one of my most favored vegetarian dishes, as you can slop it on a salad, rest it on some rice, or eat it solo. It can also replace any starchy veg to balance your plate—a potent protein with complementary (and healthy) carbs....

INGREDIENTS:

1 cup French lentils or green lentils

3 cups water

2 tablespoons extra virgin olive oil

2 garlic cloves, minced

1 large yellow onion, thinly sliced

1 cup pepper (bell, long green, or shisito), small dice

¼ teaspoon chipotle or crushed red pepper flakes

½ cup water

1 teaspoon salt

½ cup cilantro leaves, loosely packed, roughly chopped

METHOD:

1. Place the lentils and 3 cups water in a small pot. Cover and bring to a boil over medium high heat. Reduce to a simmer and cook, covered, for 10 minutes. Drain using a fine-mesh strainer.

2. In a large pan, heat the olive oil over medium heat and add the garlic, onion, pepper, and chipotle flakes. Cook until vegetables are soft, stirring occasionally, about 10 minutes. Add the finished lentils, remaining ½ cup water, and salt and cook for another 10 minutes. Toss with the cilantro.

STEFANIE'S NOTES

Store in the fridge for up to three days or freeze for up to three months. When reheating, add a little water.

PAIR WITH:

Greek Goddess Salad (page 251)
Steamed rice (cooked as per package)
or
Crunchy Cabbage Slaw (page 255)
Chicken and Rice Soup (page 266)

Cowgirl Chili   SERVES 4 TO 6

While my husband complains that I always put too much stuff in my chili, everyone else seems to love it. Packed with wholesome goodness in the beans, plus veg, healthy fat, and spice, this dish is medicinally delish. Speaking of spice, when testing, we added way too much, nearly blowing a hole in my mouth (thus the name Cowgirl Chili), but much to my surprise, everyone still loved it. The spice has been sliced, but add more if you want to electrify your senses and decrease inflammation. Eat alone with a dollop of plain yogurt or sour cream and sliced avocado, as the "meat" of a burrito or as a little dip on a chip.

INGREDIENTS:

  2 tablespoons extra virgin olive oil

  1 small red onion, thinly sliced

  3 garlic cloves, chopped

  2 teaspoons ground cumin

  1 teaspoon chili powder, medium spice

  ½ cup red bell pepper, small dice

  1 small zucchini, cut into quarter-moons

  1 small yellow squash, cut into quarter-moons

  1 15-ounce can pinto beans, drained and rinsed

  1 15-ounce can black beans, drained and rinsed

  1 15-ounce can diced tomatoes

  1 8-ounce can tomato paste

  ½ cup cilantro leaves, loosely packed, roughly chopped

  Salt, to taste

METHOD:

1. In a large pot, heat the olive oil over medium heat. Add the onion, garlic, cumin, and chili powder and sauté until tender, about 3 to 5 minutes. Add the bell pepper, zucchini, and yellow squash, mix well, and cook for another 5 minutes.

2. Add the beans, diced tomatoes, and tomato paste to the pot and stir well. Cover and simmer for 10 minutes. Remove the cover and simmer for another 10 minutes.

3. Add the cilantro and gently mix. Season with salt to taste.

STEFANIE'S NOTES

Store in the fridge for up to three days or freeze for up to three months.

PAIR WITH:

  Cheesy Bok Choy Caesar Salad (page 254)

  Curried Sweet Potato Mash (page 270)

Thaied-Up Tempeh

SERVES 4

Tempeh has a distinct flavor so many don't dare to try it, but team it up with some serious sauce and it's sure to delight. It is one of the least-processed forms of soy outside whole soybeans themselves (such as edamame), so if you want the benefits of this bean, say good-bye to the highly processed soy protein isolates and textured vegetable protein that pump packaged food with power and try some tempeh.

INGREDIENTS:

2 packages tempeh

3 tablespoon coconut or vegetable oil

2 garlic cloves, minced

1 tablespoon minced fresh ginger root

2 large scallions, thinly sliced

1 15-ounce can coconut milk

1 teaspoon honey

2 tablespoons tamari or soy sauce

2 tablespoons fresh lime juice

½ cup cilantro leaves, loosely packed, roughly chopped

METHOD:

1. Cut each slab of tempeh horizontally into three even pieces. Then cut each "square" in half on the diagonal, making triangles.

2. In a large sauté pan, heat the coconut oil over medium heat. Place the tempeh in the pan and cook until golden, 2–3 minutes on each side. Remove from the pan and set aside. Immediately add the garlic, ginger, and scallions and cook for 3 minutes, tossing occasionally.

3. Add the coconut milk, honey, and tamari. Bring to a boil over high heat, then reduce to a simmer and add the tempeh. Spoon the sauce over the tempeh, cover the pan, and cook for 15 minutes, regularly basting with a spoon.

4. Garnish with the lime juice and cilantro.

The longer the tempeh sits in the sauce, the more flavor it will have. So save some for a "leftover lunch." Store in the fridge for up to three days. Also, if you are not a fan of tempeh, you can substitute 1 pound of fish (your preference) or chicken (white or dark meat).

PAIR WITH:

Wilted Greens (page 258)
Steamed rice (cooked as per package)

Untraditional Egg Salad   SERVES 4

While I love the idea of egg salad—a quick, potentially nourishing grab, it is typically a no-go food for me because of the all-too-common gobs of mayonnaise. One morning, with a couple of hard-boiled eggs in a bowl, I added some avocado and mashed away. The result? A untraditional egg salad. So, for whatever meal you please, even for a snack, this dish is delicious and nutritious. And with no mayo.

INGREDIENTS:

4 large hard-boiled eggs, roughly chopped
1 avocado, soft but fresh, medium dice
2 teaspoons fresh lemon juice
1 small garlic clove, minced
2 large scallions, thinly sliced
½ cup flat-leaf parsley, loosely packed, roughly chopped
Salt, to taste
Freshly ground black pepper, to taste

METHOD:

1. Fill small pot with water, gently add eggs, and bring to a boil, uncovered, on medium high. Remove from heat and let sit for about 15 minutes. Slightly crack eggs and place in cold water bath to cool. Then peel.

2. In a medium bowl, mash the eggs with fork. Add the avocado and continue to mash. Add the lemon juice, garlic, scallions, and parsley and mix well. Season with salt and pepper to taste.

STEFANIE'S NOTES

Great the day after, but don't keep longer than that.

PAIR WITH:

Cauliflower Cheese Soup (page 264)
Grainy bread

Fish Tacos   SERVES 4 TO 6

Who doesn't love a good fish taco—so easy to make, plus fun for kids and grown-ups to assemble. These are pretty zesty and uncomplicated, but feel free to layer on more flavor with fixins like guacamole, plain yogurt or sour cream, and a sprinkle of cheese. If you or your kids prefer the plain, let the fish stand alone as your "fish stick" and dunk it in a little ketchup.

FOR FISH:

1½ pounds flounder fillets or other white flaky fish
Juice of 1 lemon, for cleaning fish
1 teaspoon salt, for cleaning fish
½ cup grapeseed oil or other vegetable oil, for frying

FOR COATING:

1 cup yellow cornmeal
½ teaspoon salt

FOR SAUCE:

½ cup plain thick yogurt such as Greek
1 tablespoon sour cream

¼ teaspoon maple syrup

3 tablespoons fresh lime juice

1 small shallot, minced

⅛ teaspoon chipotle or crushed red pepper flakes

½ teaspoon ground cumin

½ cup flat-leaf parsley, loosely packed, roughly chopped

FOR ASSEMBLY:

6 soft corn tortillas

2 cups shredded romaine lettuce

½ cup salsa

METHOD:

1. Clean the fish with the lemon juice and salt, rinse under cold water, and pat dry with a paper towel. Cut into bite-size chunks.

2. In a large sauté pan, heat the grapeseed oil over medium-high heat.

3. Mix the cornmeal and salt. Dredge the fish in the coating, shaking off the excess cornmeal. Then pan-fry the fish in the heated grapeseed oil, 2 to 3 minutes per side. When done, place the chunks on a plate covered with a paper towel (to drain the excess oil).

4. To make the sauce, combine the yogurt, sour cream, maple syrup, lime juice, shallot, chipotle flakes, cumin, and parsley in a small bowl and mix well.

5. For taco assembly, warm the corn tortillas in a toaster oven or in a dry sauté pan. Layer the warmed tortillas with lettuce, two or three pieces of fish, a heaping tablespoon of sauce, and a dollop of salsa.

PAIR WITH:

Skillet Broccoli (page 256)

Acorn Squash Chips (page 272)

Vegetable-Smothered Halibut   SERVES 4

Each summer my family ventures to Maine for a little vacation. We pass time with my colleague and friend John Bagnulo and his family, whose house, built into a hillside, is surrounded by lush food-bearing gardens, chickens, and goats. Of course much of our time is spent cooking and eating. When we arrived one summer a side of fish was waiting with bowls of vegetables, from garlic and onions to tomatoes, zucchini, and kale. My approach was to sauté the veg, smother the fish, and bake it all in the oven. John, also an avid cook and eater, was stunned. He never knew it could be that simple. . . .

FOR FISH:

1½ pounds halibut fillets (or any fish), 1½ to 2 inches thick

Juice of 1 lemon, for cleaning fish

1 teaspoon salt, for cleaning fish

FOR VEGETABLES:

3 tablespoons extra virgin olive oil

3 garlic cloves, minced

1 large leek, top and bottom trimmed, cut in half lengthwise and thoroughly cleaned, thinly sliced

1 small carrot, julienned

1 small yellow squash, small dice

½ teaspoon ground cumin

½ teaspoon salt

2 cups shredded kale

½ cup flat-leaf parsley, loosely packed, roughly chopped

2 tablespoons fresh lemon juice

METHOD:

1. Preheat the oven to 350°F.

2. To clean the fish, wash it with the lemon juice and salt, rinse it under cold water, and pat it dry with a paper towel. Place the whole fish fillet in a baking dish.

3. In a large sauté pan, heat the olive oil over medium heat. Add the garlic, leek, carrot, squash, cumin, and salt. Cook for 5 minutes, stirring regularly.

4. Add the kale, parsley, and lemon juice and toss, cooking for another 5 minutes.

5. When the vegetables are done, smother the fish with the mixture and cover with foil. Bake for 10 minutes. Remove the foil and bake for another 10 minutes or until the internal temperature on the fish reaches 145°F.

STEFANIE'S NOTES

Great the day after for a "leftover lunch" or even an easy dinner, but don't keep longer than that.

PAIR WITH:

Greens and Beans Salad (page 252)
Pesto Pasta (page 273)

Teriyaki Salmon   SERVES 4

I love teriyaki, but it is way too sweet. So I created my own. And as my culinary partner in crime, Rebecca Katz, says, "Where is the YUM factor?" Well, the salty crashes into sweet with perfect precision. Add a little garlic and ginger and you have a tasty teriyaki that is light and goes with any kind of fleshy food, vegetables, and can even be drizzled on a bowl of rice.

FOR FISH:

1½ pounds salmon fillets (or any meaty fish), 1½ to 2 inches thick

Juice of 1 lemon, for cleaning fish

1 teaspoon salt, for cleaning fish

FOR TERIYAKI:

¼ cup tamari or soy sauce

5 tablespoons maple syrup

3 garlic cloves, minced

1 tablespoon minced fresh ginger root

METHOD:

1. Preheat the oven to 350°F.

2. Clean the fish with the lemon juice and salt, rinse it under cold water, and pat it dry with a paper towel. Place the whole fish fillet in a baking dish.

3. In a small pot, combine the tamari, maple syrup, garlic, and ginger. Simmer until it bubbles, about 5 minutes. Remove from the heat and set aside.

4. With a fork or your clean fingers, poke holes in the flesh of the fish, then pour the sauce on top, making sure to cover the fish. For medium to well-done fish, bake for 18 to 20 minutes, or until the internal temperature on the fish reaches at least 145°F, then turn the oven to broil and cook for another 3 minutes.

STEFANIE'S NOTES

Great the day after for a "leftover lunch" or even an easy dinner, but don't keep longer than that. However, the sauce will keep for about a week in an airtight container in the fridge.

PAIR WITH:

Must-Have Miso Soup (page 263)

Vegetable Fried Rice (page 277)

Macadamia Monkfish   SERVES 4

Monkfish, often called poor man's lobster, is fit for any king as far as I am con-
cerned. While far less costly than its crustacean counterpart, monkfish is tender
yet meaty, and when cooked in this Hawaiian-inspired sauce, it melts in your
mouth.

FOR FISH:

    1½ pounds monkfish (or any white flaky or meaty fish)

    Juice of 1 lemon, for cleaning fish

    1 teaspoon salt, for cleaning fish

FOR COATING:

    ½ cup ground macadamia nuts

    ½ cup cilantro leaves, loosely packed, finely chopped

    ½ teaspoon salt

    ½ cup coconut milk

METHOD:

1. Preheat the oven to 350°F.

2. If the thin outer membrane has not been removed from the fish, do so with your clean hands by easing your fingers between the membrane and the flesh of the fish, tearing away the thin sheath. Then clean the fish by rubbing it with the lemon juice and salt, rinsing it under cold water, and patting it dry. Place the whole fish fillet in a baking dish.

3. Combine the nuts, cilantro, and salt in a food processor and pulse until semifine, or you can simply chop them with a knife.

4. Add the coconut milk to the baking dish, then cover the fillet with the nut coating using a spoon (you can also press it into the fish with your clean hands). Cover the baking dish with foil and bake for 10 minutes, then remove the foil and bake for another 20 minutes or until the internal temperature on the fish reaches 145°F.

Great the day after for a "leftover lunch" or even an easy dinner, but don't keep longer than that.

PAIR WITH:

Wilted Greens (page 258)
Curried Sweet Potato Mash (page 270)

Baked Buffalo Wings with Creamy Ranch   SERVES 4

My mom has been making some mean chicken wings for as long as I can remember. They were a family favorite growing up and are still hanging in years later. She often makes them for large family dinners, where eleven of us gather to share a meal. The five grandkids have caught on to the wing factor, and between them and my father, few are left by dinnertime. So now my mom hides them—smart woman! This is my twist on her creation. They are also super delish to munch on during your favorite football game....

FOR WINGS:

2 pounds chicken wings
Juice of 1 lemon, for cleaning chicken
1 teaspoon salt, for cleaning chicken
2 teaspoons paprika
1 teaspoon black pepper
2 teaspoons onion powder
4 tablespoons extra virgin olive oil
1 teaspoon salt
¼ cup fresh lemon juice

FOR CREAMY RANCH:

½ cup Greek yogurt
¼ cup sour cream

1 teaspoon fresh lemon juice

1 garlic clove, minced

1 tablespoon dried dill

½ teaspoon onion powder

¼ teaspoon salt

METHOD:

1. Clean the chicken wings with lemon juice and salt, rinse them under cold water, and pat them dry with a paper towel. Place the wings in a large mixing bowl with the paprika, pepper, onion powder, olive oil, and the remaining salt and lemon juice. Mix well to evenly coat all of the wings. Cover the bowl and marinate for 1 hour (or up to 24 hours) in the fridge.

2. When you are ready to cook the wings, preheat the oven to 350°F. Remove the chicken from the fridge and let it sit at room temperature while the oven is preheating.

3. Place the wings on a parchment-lined baking sheet in a single layer and bake for 45 minutes. Flip the wings and bake for another 15 to 20 minutes.

4. Combine the ranch ingredients in a small bowl and mix well. Serve with the wings.

PAIR WITH:

Crunchy Cabbage Slaw (page 255)

Butternut Squash Risotto (page 275)

Cornmeal-Crusted Chicken Cutlets   SERVES 4

My son Hunter has a fairly limited palate. He was plagued with feeding problems in his early years (see sidebar, "Respecting Funny Little Eating Habits," page 212), so eating has always been a bit of a challenge. Like most kids with a limited culinary repertoire, he enjoys his chicken nuggets. And I'll be damned if he's gonna eat chicken out of a box all of the time. This is my manifestation of the mainstream nugget or tender. And Hunter loves them, most of the time. Oh, and if you like any kind of breaded bird dish like chicken Parmesan, use these cutlets as your foundation.

FOR CHICKEN:

   1½ pounds boneless chicken cutlets, about ¼–½-inch thick

   Juice of 1 lemon, for cleaning chicken

   1 teaspoon salt, for cleaning chicken

FOR COATING:

   1 cup extra virgin olive oil (to coat the chicken)

   1 cup yellow cornmeal

   2 tablespoons dried oregano

   2 tablespoons dried basil

   1 teaspoon salt, plus more to taste

FOR FRYING:

   ½ cup grapeseed oil or other vegetable oil, for frying

METHOD:

   1. Clean the chicken with the lemon juice and salt, rinse it under cold water, and pat it dry with a paper towel.

   2. Place the chicken in a medium bowl and add the olive oil to coat. On a large plate, combine the cornmeal, oregano, basil, and remaining salt. Mix well.

   3. In a large sauté pan, heat oil over medium heat. Dredge each piece of chicken in the cornmeal mixture, shaking off the excess, then place the pieces in the pan and cook until golden, 3 to 4 minutes per side or until the internal temperature on the chicken reaches 165°F.

   4. When done, place the cutlets on a plate covered with a paper towel to drain off the excess oil. Season with salt to taste.

These cutlets are definitely durable. They can be stored in the fridge for up to three days and yes, you can even freeze them for up to three months (but if you are planning to do so, I suggest partially cooking them prior to freezing so they don't give you dry mouth when defrosted and reheated, whether in a pan with some oil or in the oven).

PAIR WITH:

Shards of Brussels with Herbed Dijon (page 257)
Naked Eggplant Parmesan (page 261)

Savory Herb-Roasted Chicken   SERVES 4

Roasting a whole chicken can seem super daunting to many—from flavoring it to cooking it. First, the trick to making the bird bust with aroma is giving it a full-body massage with an herby rub. Once you do that, pop it in the oven (lower heat for a little longer does wonders), occasionally bathing it in its juices. Sometimes your soul just needs a good roasted chicken.

FOR CHICKEN:

1 whole chicken, 4 to 5 pounds
Juice of 1 lemon, to clean chicken
1 teaspoon salt, to clean chicken
1 large yellow onion

FOR HERB RUB:

½ cup extra virgin olive oil
2 teaspoons salt
4 garlic cloves
1 cup flat-leaf parsley, loosely packed

2 tablespoons fresh oregano, loosely packed

2 tablespoons fresh rosemary, loosely packed

1 tablespoon fresh thyme leaves

METHOD:

1. Preheat the oven to 375°F; make sure that the oven rack is centered in the oven.

2. Remove the neck from inside the chicken cavity and discard. Clean the chicken with the lemon juice and salt, rinse it under cold water, and pat it dry with a paper towel. Place the chicken in a roasting pan or 3- to 4-inch deep large baking dish. Quarter the onion (you do not have to peel it) and place it inside the cavity.

3. To make the rub, combine the olive oil, salt, garlic, and herbs in a food processor and purée into a paste. Use your hands to create a space between the skin of the chicken and the body. Place some of the mixture in that space as well as all over the skin of the chicken.

4. Place the baking dish in the center of the oven rack and cook until the internal temperature reads 165°F, regularly basting the chicken until golden brown, about 1 hour, 15 minutes.

STEFANIE'S NOTES

If you have leftover meat, remove it from the carcass and toss it in a salad for a "leftover lunch."

PAIR WITH:

Kale Ratatouille (page 259)

Zucchini Latkes (page 271)

Mon Frères Turkey Meatballs   SERVES 4 TO 6

My brother loves to cook. He often shares his culinary secrets with me, especially when it comes cooking technique or spicing. And most of the time, I'm all ears.

One of my favorites is his meatball approach. Instead of the typical pan-frying, he briefly bakes the meatballs, keeping the moisture in, then plops them into the heated sauce. If you don't want turkey, try them with ground chicken or red meat. Equally good . . .

FOR MEATBALLS:

  2 pounds ground turkey
  1 large egg
  ¼ cup cornmeal or bread crumbs
  2 tablespoons Dijon mustard
  4 garlic cloves, minced
  2 tablespoons dried oregano
  2 teaspoons salt

FOR SAUCE:

  2 tablespoons extra virgin olive oil
  4 cloves minced garlic
  1 large onion, small dice
  2 28-ounce cans crushed tomatoes
  2 medium sprigs fresh rosemary
  Salt to taste (optional)

METHOD:

  1. Preheat the oven to 350°F.

  2. In a large bowl, combine the meatball ingredients. Mix thoroughly with your hands, form the mixture into balls (the size of a golf ball), and place them on a lightly oiled or parchment-lined baking sheet. Bake for 15 minutes.

  3. To make the sauce, in a large pot, heat the olive oil over medium heat and sauté the garlic and onion for 3 minutes, tossing regularly. Add the tomatoes and rosemary, cover the pot, and simmer for 8 to 10 minutes.

  4. When the meatballs are done, remove them from the oven. Using tongs, place them one by one in the pot with the sauce. Cook over low heat,

covered, for another 30 minutes. Remove the rosemary sprigs and discard. Salt to taste if needed.

STEFANIE'S NOTES

Ground turkey meat can be very sticky. Keep your hands lightly coated with olive oil when mixing meat and forming into meatballs. The finished meatballs can be stored in the fridge for up to three days or frozen for up to three months.

PAIR WITH:

Cheesy Bok Choy Caesar Salad (page 254)
Cooked pasta

Asian-Marinated Flank Steak

SERVES 4 TO 6

This marinade is mouthwatering. It's like a sweet-and-sour sauce with a splash of spice that dazzles any dish whether steak, poultry, or fish. All recipes stem from some sort of inspiration, and this one was based on an Asian-style barbecue sauce that was featured in a magazine decades ago. After I tried it in my own kitchen, satisfying the more simplistic of cooks was a must. So I reinvented this bursting-with-flavor barbecue.

FOR STEAK:

2 pounds flank steak
Juice of 1 lemon, to clean meat
1 teaspoon salt, to clean meat

FOR MARINADE:

¾ cup Thai red chili paste, Thai Kitchen brand

1½ cups mirin

6 tablespoons tamari or soy sauce

12 garlic cloves, minced

6 tablespoons minced fresh ginger root

½ cup sesame oil (light in color)

4 large scallions, thinly sliced

1 cup cilantro leaves, loosely packed, roughly chopped

METHOD:

1. To clean the steak, wash it with the lemon juice and salt, rinse it under cold water, and pat it dry with a paper towel.

2. Combine the marinade ingredients in a large bowl and mix well.

3. Portion half of the marinade and place in a heavy-duty zip-lock bag with the steak and marinate for at least 1 hour in the fridge (or overnight). Set the remaining marinade aside in an airtight container in the fridge.

4. Thirty minutes before cooking, remove the marinating steak from the fridge and let it come to room temperature. Just before cooking, remove the steak from the bag and discard (with marinade).

5. In a small pot, warm the remaining marinade on low heat.

6. For medium steak, cook 5 minutes on each side whether grilling, cooking on a griddle or in a skillet, or broiling in the oven. For more well-done steak, cook it longer. When the steak is finished, let it sit for 5 minutes. Slice the steak and top it with the marinade.

STEFANIE'S NOTES

Great as a "leftover lunch" tossed on top of a salad or for an easy dinner a day or two after, but don't keep it past that.

PAIR WITH:

Skillet Broccoli (page 256)

Butternut Squash Risotto (page 275)

Montauk Meat Loaf

This is for all the meat-loving Montaukians who appreciate the gifts from the local sea but need a good hunk of meat once in a while. It's a family-and-friends favorite, especially with a good baked potato or some mash, on those chilly and ghost town–like days when we all gather to feast by a fire. If you don't do cow, try it with poultry.

INGREDIENTS:

- 1½ pounds lean ground beef
- 1 tablespoon extra virgin olive oil
- 1 large egg
- 1 tablespoon Dijon mustard
- 1 6-ounce can tomato paste, 2 tablespoons reserved
- 2 garlic cloves, minced
- ½ small yellow onion, small dice
- 1 tablespoon minced fresh oregano leaves
- 1 tablespoon minced fresh rosemary leaves
- ¼ cup yellow cornmeal or bread crumbs
- 2 teaspoons salt

METHOD:

1. Preheat the oven to 350°F.

2. In a large bowl, combine the ground beef, olive oil, egg, mustard, all but 2 tablespoons of the tomato paste, garlic, onion, oregano, rosemary, cornmeal, and salt and mix with clean hands until combined.

3. In a baking dish, form the meat into a 2-inch-high loaf and generously coat with the remaining 2 tablespoons of tomato paste. Cover the dish with foil and bake for 45 minutes. Remove the foil and bake for another 30 minutes or until the internal temperature on the meat reaches 160°F.

Great as a "leftover lunch," solo, or on a sandwich. Also perfect for an easy dinner a day or two after, though don't keep it past that.

PAIR WITH:
Shards of Brussels with Herbed Dijon (page 257)
Curried Sweet Potato Mash (page 270)

To-Die-For Desserts

Cooking intuitively is my thing. So you won't be surprised when I tell you that all of my measuring spoons and cups that were trashed when my boys were little (something for them to play with) were never replaced until *What the Fork* recipe testing was staring me in the face.

You see, the only time that I actually measure anything is when I am testing recipes or baking. And I never bake because I suck at it—the exacting nature is equal to locking me in a cage. So consider me a half-assed baker aiming for sweets that allow for a little laziness. If my measurements are a tad off, it's no biggie. I don't pair desserts with anything other than a cool cup of water or a glorious glass of milk (whatever your preference, dairy or nondairy).

Jack's Banana Ice Cream
Salty Caramel Apples
Almond Butter and Jelly Cookies
Maple Pecan Chip Cookies
Carrot Cupcakes

Jack's Banana Ice Cream   SERVES 4

Not only is this an all-time family favorite but every client and student of mine is blown away by the simplicity and deliciousness of this recipe. My son Jack likes to play around with this creamy pleasure, adding everything from cinnamon to chocolate chips and nuts, though he has pretty much settled on this version as his favorite.

INGREDIENTS:

2 large bananas (not overripe), peeled, cut into quarters, and frozen

2 tablespoons coconut or other milk

2 teaspoons minced fresh ginger root

½ tablespoon maple syrup, or to taste

METHOD:

Combine all ingredients in a food processor and purée until creamy, about 5 minutes. Taste; if it is not sweet enough (sweetness depends on the bananas' ripeness), add more maple syrup to taste.

STEFANIE'S NOTES

Enjoy immediately. If you wait to eat it, the bananas will turn.

Salty Caramel Apples   MAKES 1 CUP CARAMEL

Any way you slice it, caramel is not health supportive. But it is darn delicious. A few years ago, fussing in my kitchen over some caramel popcorn creation, I morphed an unremarkable recipe into this holy-cow caramel. Twisting the recipe, adding a little coarse sea salt, and tossing it atop some green or red apples made something ordinary absolutely outstanding.

INGREDIENTS:

1 stick unsalted butter

1 cup dark brown sugar

¼ cup brown rice syrup

½ teaspoon pure vanilla extract

¼ teaspoon baking soda

2 teaspoons rock sea salt

4 large apples, sliced

METHOD:

1. In a small pot, melt the butter over medium heat. Add the brown sugar and brown rice syrup and whisk. Bring to a slow boil over medium-high heat, then reduce to a simmer.

2. Add the vanilla and baking soda and whisk until mixed well, at which point the caramel will bubble. Remove from the heat immediately to let caramel settle (about 2 minutes). Stir in salt.

3. Either serve warm with apples or transfer to a glass container to cool, then store in the fridge.

STEFANIE'S NOTES

Forget the apples and eat on top of frozen yogurt or ice cream. It's even good solo. Store in the fridge for up to one week.

Almond Butter and Jelly Cookies
MAKES 12 LARGE COOKIES

An almond butter and jelly sandwich in a cookie? You can't beat that. Or use peanut butter if you prefer. Great as a dessert but also as a pick-me-up snack during the day, as any nut butter (if not laden with sugar and trans fat) is packed with nutrition. Be sure to have a glass of liquid handy, as this cookie loves mouth rooftops.

INGREDIENTS:

½ cup almond butter

⅓ cup safflower or sunflower oil

½ cup maple syrup

1 teaspoon pure vanilla extract

¼ teaspoon salt

1½ cups flour (whole wheat, spelt, or gluten-free)

½ cup fruit preserves, any flavor

METHOD:

1. Preheat the oven to 350°F.

2. In a large bowl, mix the almond butter, safflower oil, maple syrup, vanilla, and salt with a wooden spoon. Add flour and mix well to form a dough.

3. To make the cookies, form golf-ball–size balls with the dough, place the balls on a lightly oiled cookie sheet, and press the dough to form a round cookie about ¼ inch thick. Using your thumb, form a groove in the center of the cookie and add 1 tablespoon of preserves; repeat until all cookies are done. Bake for 20 minutes.

STEFANIE'S NOTES

Store in an airtight container in a cool, dry place for three to five days or in the fridge or freezer for up to three months.

Maple-Pecan Chip Cookies   MAKES 18 TO 24 COOKIES

Everybody needs a melt-in-your-mouth cookie, and this is my all-time favorite with its crumbly goodness. It's great as a grab-and-go snack or crumbled on top of some yogurt (preferably plain) like any granola. Keep 'em in the fridge or freezer for the ultimate crunch factor. Also, use the batter (without the chips) as a crust for any crumble. Versatile and victorious.

INGREDIENTS:

2 cups rolled oats, ground to coarse meal in a food processor

2 cups pecans, ground to coarse meal in a food processor

1 cup oat flour

1 cup brown rice flour

¾ cup maple syrup

1 cup safflower or sunflower oil

4 teaspoons pure vanilla extract

¼ teaspoon sea salt

1 teaspoon ground cinnamon

1 cup semisweet chocolate chips (optional)

METHOD:

1. Preheat the oven to 350°F.

2. Combine all ingredients in a large bowl and mix thoroughly.

3. Form the dough into golf-ball–size balls with your clean hands and press them onto a parchment-lined cookie sheet until they are about ⅛ inch thick. Bake for 15 minutes. Let them cool on the cookie sheet before removing (otherwise they will crumble).

STEFANIE'S NOTES

If you don't like chocolate, lose the chips. Store in an airtight container in a cool, dry place for three to five days or in the fridge or freezer for up to three months.

Carrot Cupcakes   MAKES 12 LARGE CUPCAKES

Never much of a cake eater, I am not a connoisseur. However, put a carrot cake in front of me and I will gobble it up—hold the raisins, make sure it's moist, and gimme a good frosting (yes, one with highly processed confectioner's sugar). This is my take on the perfect carrot cake. Without the frosting, these cupcakes can "moonlight" as a morning munch or even a healthy daytime snack.

FOR CUPCAKES:

1 cup maple syrup

1 cup grated carrots

1 teaspoon ground cinnamon

1 teaspoon ground nutmeg

½ teaspoon ground cloves

¼ cup coconut oil

¼ cup apple butter or applesauce

1 teaspoon pure vanilla extract

1 cup unsweetened soy milk

2 cups flour (spelt, whole wheat, or gluten-free)

2 teaspoons baking soda

¾ cup chopped walnuts

FOR FROSTING:

8 ounces cream cheese

½ cup unsalted butter, softened

½ teaspoon pure vanilla extract

Pinch of ground cinnamon

¼ cup plus 2 tablespoons confectioners' sugar

METHOD:

1. Preheat the oven to 350°F.

2. In a large saucepan, combine the maple syrup, carrots, cinnamon, nutmeg, cloves, coconut oil, apple butter, vanilla, and soy milk and bring to a slow boil over medium-high heat, then remove from heat.

3. In a large bowl, mix the flour, baking soda, and walnuts. Add the liquid ingredients and mix well.

4. Pour the batter into muffin cups (using paper liners if necessary) and bake for 20 minutes.

5. Combine the frosting ingredients in a bowl and beat with a hand mixer (or other). Let the cupcakes cool before frosting.

STEFANIE'S NOTES

Store unfrosted cupcakes in the fridge for up to one week or freeze for up to three months.

One Last Word

Throughout my years of practicing with clients one-on-one, they have consistently urged me to get my message out there. They said that people needed my food and nutrition guidance in my no-nonsense kinda way.

Well, thank you, clients, as you all gave me the impetus to pursue *What the Fork*. And with it, I hope I have accomplished my goal—reaching a larger audience with this critical information, as well as giving readers the tools to actually make the changes I am talking about, even if very small.

While I wish I could be that little birdie sitting on everyone's shoulder through this food lifestyle change (or whatever you want to call it), I can't be everywhere all at once (though sometimes I like to think I can). So let *What the Fork* be your guide—you now have the knowledge and skills to start shifting your paradigm.

Oh, and one last thing—please turn your ears off to most everything you hear or see in the media about food and nutrition unless from a truly credible expert; instead call on unsensationalized information in the resources provided in the book and listed in Appendix E, "Redeemable Resources." Definitely ditch the diet fads because in the end, they won't do you much good. If you have health issues, and diet can be used as a part of your prescription, seek the care of a credible nutrition practitioner (with some combination of letters like MS, RDN, PhD, CN, CNS, and CDN, and LDN after their name) to help you get from A to Z.

What the Fork is your blueprint to rebuild your foundation with food. And hopefully you enjoyed reading it and using it as much as I relished writing it!

The Who's Who in Big Food and the Good Guys They "Ate"

Herein is the handful of large food companies that own others, whether medium or small (and all of their brands). Many if not most of the products you consume today are inclusive. While I have aimed to provide you with the most updated comprehensive list, please note that the sale and acquisition of food companies is in constant motion. Peruse the list and you will most likely find many of your brands here, good or not so good.

BIG FOOD	COMMON BRAND NAMES
AdvancePierre Foods LLC	Fast Fixin', Barber Foods, Pierre Drive Thru, Pierre Signatures, Big Az, Hot n' Ready, Pierre, The Pub
Agri-Mark	Agrimark, Cabot, McCadam
Agropur Cooperative	Agropur Signature, Allegro, ANCO, Island Farms, La Lacteo, Natrel, OKA, Olympic, Quebon, Schroeder, Sealtest, Trega Foods, Vaudreuil, Ultra'milk, Yoplait (sold under a distribution agreement)
American Crystal Sugar Co.	Crystal sugar
American Foods Group LLC	American Foods Group, Dakota Brand, Heartland, Long Prairie Packing, O'Brien's, Sheboygan, Skylark
Anheuser Busch InBev	Anheuser World Select, American Red, Azteca, Bacardi Specialty Malt Beverages, Bare Knuckle Stout, Becks, Bud, Budweiser, Busch, Chelada Bud, Goose Island, Hurricane, King

BIG FOOD	COMMON BRAND NAMES
Anheuser Busch InBev (cont'd.)	Cobra, Land Shark Lager, Michelob, Natural Ice, Natural Light, O'Doul's, Redbridge, Rolling Rock, Rock Green Light, Rio Cristal, Shock Top, Skol, Stella Artois, Stone Mill Pale Ale, Tequiza, Ziegenbock
B&G Foods Inc.	Accent, Baker's Joy, B&G Condiments, Brer Rabbit, Cream of Wheat, Crock-Pot Seasonings, Devonsheer, Don Pepino, Emeril's, Grandma Molasses, Joan of Arc, Las Palmas, Maple Grove Farms, Molly McButter, Mrs. Dash, New York Style, Old London, Ortega, Polaner, Regina, Slafani, Sugar Twin, Trappey's, TrueNorth, Underwood, Vermont Maid, Wright's
Beam Inc.	Jim Beam, Maker's Mark, Sauza, Pinnacle, Courvoisier, Canadian Club, Teacher's, Basil Hayden's, Knob Creek, Skinny Girl
Bimbo Bakeries USA	Arnold, Bimbo, Boboli, Brownberry, Entenmann's, Francisco, Freihofer's, Ideal, Marinela, Mrs. Baird's, Old Country Bread, Oroweat, Plus Vita, Pullman, Stroehmann, Thomas', Tia Rosa
Borden Dairy Co.	Milk Products LP, Borden, Chattanooga Dairy, Coburg Dairy, Cream O'Weber, Dairy Fresh, Dairy Fresh of Louisiana, Dairymens, Flav O-Rich, H. Meyer, Sinton, U.C. Milk (dba Goldenrod Dairy), Velda Farms
Brown-Forman Corp.	Bel Arbor, Bonterra, Canadian Mist, Chambord, Early Times, el Jimador, Fetzer, Finlandia, Five Rivers, Gentleman Jack, Herradura, Jack Daniel's, Jekel, Korbel, Little Black Dress, Old Forester, Pepe Lopez, Sanctuary, Sonoma-Cutrer, Southern Comfort, Tuaca, Woodford Reserve
California Dairies Inc.	California Dairies, Challenge Dairy Products, Danish Creamery
Campbell Soup Co.	Arnott's, Bolthouse Farms, Campbell's, Chunky, Franco-American, Godiva, Goldfish, Healthy Request, Hungry-Man, Pace, Pepperidge Farm, Plum Organics, Prego, Royco, SpaghettiOs, Swanson, Supper Bakes, V8 Vegetable Juice, Wolfgang Puck
Canada Bread Co. (Maple Leaf Foods 90 percent ownership)	Burns, California Goldminer, Hygrade, Nutriwhip, Olafson's Baking Company, Prime Turkey, Shopsy's Tenderflake, Maison-Cousin, Dempsters, Olivieri, New York Bakery Co.

BIG FOOD	COMMON BRAND NAMES
Cargill Inc. (see the following diagram for joint alliances with organic food producers)	Cargill Beef, Cargill Case Ready, Cargill Kitchen Solutions, Cargill Pork, Cargill Salt, Cargill Value Added Meats Food Service, Cargill Value Added Meats Retail, Cargill Cocoa and Chocolate North America, Cargill Corn Milling North America, Cargill Dressings, Sauces and Oils, Cargill Malt, Cargill Specialty Seeds and Oils, Cargill Texturizing Solutions, Horizon Milling
Chiquita	Chiquita, Fresh Express
Chobani Inc.	Chobani, Chobani Champions
Coca-Cola Co.	Abbey Well, Aquarius, Barq's, Blak, Bright & Early, Canada Dry, Carver's, Citra, Coca-Cola, Coke, Dasani, Diet Coke, Fanta, Five Alive, Flavor Rage, Fresca, Fruitopia, Full Throttle, Georgia, Glacéau vitaminwater, Hi-C, Honest, Illy Issimo, Inca Cola, Manzana Mia, Mello Yello, Minute Maid, Mr. Pibb, Nestea, Northern Neck, Odwalla, Powerade, Red Flash, Schweppes, Seagram's, Simply, Sprite, Surge, Tab, Vault
Colgate-Palmolive Co.	Colgate, Palmolive, Soft Soap, Irish Spring, Murphy's, Swavitel, Ajaj, Lady Speed Stick, Speed Stick, Fabuloso, Hill's Prescription Diet, Hill's Science Diet
ConAgra Foods Inc.	Angela Mia, Act II, Andy Capp's, Armour, Banquet, Beatrice, Bloomfield Bakers, Blue Bonnet, Chef Boyardee, Country Pride, County Line, David, Decker, Eckrich, Egg Beaters, Fleischmann's, Gilroy, Golden Cuisine, Gulden, Healthy Choice, Hebrew National, Hunt's, Hunt's Snack Pack, Kid Cuisine, Knott's Berry Farm, La Choy, Lamb-Weston, Libby's, Lightlife, Louis Kemp, Lovin Oven, Manwich, Marie Callender's, Orville Redenbacher's, Pam, Parkay, Pemmican, Peter Pan, Rakorp (private label organic foods), Reddi-Wip, Ro-Tel, Rosarita, Snack Pack, Singleton, Slim Jim, Swift Premium, Swiss Miss, Van Camp's, Wesson
Cott Corp.	Ben Shaw's, Cott, Clear Choice, Fruit Refreshers, Orient Emporium Tea Co., So Clear, Stars & Stripes, Vess, Vintage, Mr. Fizz, Top Pop, City Club, Red Rain, Red Rooster, Royal Crown, Throwdown, Aftershock
CROPP Cooperative/ Organic Valley	Organic Valley

BIG FOOD	COMMON BRAND NAMES
Dairy Farmers of America	Borden, Breakstone's, Cache Valley, Cass-Clay Creamery, Falfurrias, Guida's, Hotel Bar, Keller's Creamery, Kemps, La Vaquita, Plugra, Sport Shake
DairyGold	Darigold
Dannon Co. Inc.	Activia, Brown Cow, DanActive, Danimals, Dan-o-nino, Dannon, Evian, Happy Family, Light & Fit, Oikos, Stonyfield Farms, YoCream
Dean Foods Co.	Alta Dena, Atlanta Dairies, Arctic Splash, Barbers, Barbe's, Berkeley Farms, Borden, Broughton, Brown Cow, Brown's Dairy, Bud's Ice Cream, Chug, Country Charm, Country Churn, Country Delite, Country Fresh, Country Love, Creamland, Dairy Fresh, Dean's, Dipzz, Foremost,* Fieldcrest, Friendship, Fruit Rush, Garelick Farms, Gandy's, Hershey's, Horizon, Hygeia, Jilbert, Land O'Lakes,* Land-O-Sun, Lehigh Valley, Liberty, Louis Trauth, Maplehurst, Mayfield, McArthur, Meadowbrook, Meadow Gold, Mile High, Mountain High, Nature's Pride, NuttyBuddy, Nurture, Oak Farms, Over The Moon, Pet, Pog Price's, Purity, Reiter, Robinson, Saunders, Schenkel's All Star, Schepps, Shenandoah's Pride, Stroh's, Swiss Dairy, Swiss Premium, TG Lee, the Organic Cow of Vermont, Tuscan, Turtle Tracks, Verifine, Viva, White Wave Silk
Del Monte Foods	Del Monte, S and W, Canine Carry Outs, Contadina, College Inn, Kibbles and Bits, MilkBone, Pup-Peroni, Meaty Bone, Snausages, Sun Fresh, Nature's Recipe, Gravy Train, Jerky Treats, 9 Lives, Meow Mix, Pounce
Diamond Foods Inc.	Diamond Culinary Nuts, Emerald Premium Nuts, Kettle Brand, Pop Secret
Dole Food Co. Inc.	Dole, Dole Classic Salad, Dole Complete Salads, Dole Fruit Bowls, Dole Lunch for One, Dole Special Blends, Dole Tropical Gold, Dole Premium Select, Wildly Nutritious
Dr Pepper Snapple Group	7UP, A&W, Canada Dry, Clamato, Country Time, Crush, Deja Blue, Diet Rite, Dr Pepper, Gini, Hawaiian Punch, Hires, IBC, Margaritaville, Mistic, Mott's, Mr and Mrs T, Nantucket Nectars, Nehi, Orangina, Peñafiel, RC Cola, ReaLemon, Rose's, Schweppes, Snapple, Squirt, Stewart's, Sundrop, Sunkist, Venom Energy, Vernors, Welch's, Yoo-hoo

BIG FOOD	COMMON BRAND NAMES
Flowers Foods Inc.	Nature's Own, Whitewheat, Cobblestone Mill, Sunbeam, Bunny, Bluebird, Mrs. Freshley's, Mi Casa, European Bakery, ButterKrust, Captain John Derst's, Evangeline Maid, Mary Jane & Friends, Aunt Hattie's, Holsum
Foremost Farms USA	127 Cheese, 1950 Cheese, Foremost Farms
Foster Farms LLC	Chicken and turkey products, Humboldt Creamery
General Mills	Basic 4, Betty Crocker, Big G cereals, Big T Burgers, Bisquick, Bugles, Cascadian Farm, Cheerios, Chex, Cinnamon Toast Crunch, Clusters, Cocoa Puffs, Cookie Crisp, Delights, Diablitos Underwood, Fiber One, Food Should Taste Good, Frescarini, Fruit Snacks, Gardetto's, Go-Gurt, Gold Medal, Golden Grahams, Green Giant, Häagen-Dazs, Hamburger Helper, Jeno's, Jus-Rol, Kix, Knack & Back, La Salteña, Larabar, Latina, Liberte, Lucky Charms, Macaroni Grill, Monsters, Mountain High, Muir Glen, Nature Valley, Oatmeal Crisp, Old El Paso, Pillsbury, Progresso, Reese's Puffs, Toaster Scrambles, Toaster Strudel, Total, Totino's, Trix, V.Pearl, Wanchai Ferry, Wheaties, Whips!, Yo-Plus, YOP, Yoplait
Gilster-Mary Lee Corp.	FasteShake, Fryin' Magic, Hospitality, Miracle Maize
Golden State Foods	Liquid products, meat products, produce, bakery (for McDonald's primarily)
Grassland Dairy	Country Cream, Fall Creek, Grassland, Wüthrich
Great Lakes Cheese Co.	Great Lakes Cheese ("natural" and processed)
H.J. Heinz Co.	Bella Rossa, Boston Market, Chef Francisco, Classico, Catelli, Complan, Dianne's, Delimex, Earth's Best, Farley's, Guloso, Heinz, Ken-L-Ration, Olivine, Ore-Ida, Orlando, Plasmon, Quality Chef Foods, Smart Ones, Starkist, TGI Friday's, TrueSoups, Wattie's, Weight Watchers, Wyler's, Vlasic
H.P. Hood Inc.	Hood, Simply Smart, Calorie Countdown, Heluva Good, Crowly, Penn Maid, Axelrod, Rosenbergers, Maggio, Brigham's, Green's, Hagan, Lactaid

BIG FOOD	COMMON BRAND NAMES
Hain Celestial Group	Arrowhead Mills, Bearitos, BluePrint, Breadshop, Casbah, DeBoles, Earth's Best, Ella's Kitchen, Hain Pure Foods, Health Valley, Imagine Foods, MaraNatha, Mountain Sun, Nile Spice, Spectrum, Sunspire, Walnut Acres, Westbrae Natural, Celestial Seasonings, Rice Dream, Soy Dream, West Soy, Boston's, Garden of Eatin', Little Bear, Shari Ann's, Terra Chips, Yves, Bell (grocery store items), Tassimo (single-serve coffee machines Ethnic Gourmet, Linda McCartney, Rosetto, Free Bird, Plainville Farms, Frutti di Bosco, Millina's Finest, Tofu Town, Greek Gods Yogurt, Hollywood, Mountain Sun, Sensible Portions
Hershey Co.	5th Avenue, Almond Joy, Amazin' Fruit Candies, Amazin' Fruit Super Fruit Breathsavers, Bubble Yum, Candies, Bridge Mixture, Brown Cow, Cadbury's Candies, Caramello, Cherry Blossom, Chipits Chocolate Chips, Chuckles, Crash Bar, Dagoba, Eat-More, Glosette, Good & Plenty, Goodies, Heath Bar, Heide, Hershey's, Hugs, Ice Breakers, Jolly Rancher, Kisses, Kit Kat, Krackel, Lowney, Luden's, Mauna Loa, Milk Duds, Mounds, Mr. Freeze, Mr. Goodbar, Nibs, NutRageous, Oh Henry!, Ovation, PayDay, Pot of Gold, Rain-Blo, Reese's, Rolo, Skor, Sour Dudes, Snacksters, Snackbarz, Special Crisp, Special Dark, Strawberry Cow, Super Bubble, Sweet Escapes, Symphony, Take5, TasteTations, Top Scotch, Twizzelators, Twizzlers, Whatchamacallit, Whoppers, Wunderbeans, York, Young & Smylie, Zagnut, Zero
Hillshire Brands	Hillshire Farm, Jimmy Dean, Ball Park, State Fair, Aidells, Gallo Salame, Sara Lee Deli, Sara Lee Desserts, Sara Lee Foodservice
Hilmar Cheese Co.	Private label cheese and dairy ingredients like whey and lactose
Hormel Foods Corp.	Black Label, Boca Grande Foods, Buffalo, by George, Carapelli, Chi-Chi's, Country Crock, Cure 81, Curemaster, Di Lusso, Dinty Moore, Don Miguel, Dona Maria, Dubuque, El Torito, Farm Fresh, Farmer John, Fast'N Easy, Herb-Ox, Herdez, Homeland, Hormel, House of Tsang, Jennie-O, Kid's Kitchen, Light & Lean, Little Sizzlers, Lloyd's, Manny's, Marrakesh Express, Mary Kitchen, MegaMex, Not-So-Sloppy-Joe, Old Smokehouse, Patak's, Peloponnese, Quick Meal, Rosa Grande, Sandwich Maker, Saag's, Skippy, Spam, Stagg, Valley Fresh, Wranglers
Hostess Brands	Ding Dongs, Donettes, Ho Hos, Hostess, Twinkies

BIG FOOD	COMMON BRAND NAMES
J.M. Smucker Co.	Adams, Crisco, Crosse & Blackwell, Dickinson's, Dunkin Donuts, Dutch Girl, Eagle Brand, Folgers, Hungry Jack, Jif, Kava, Knott's Berry Farm, Laura Scudder's, Martha White, Magnolia, Mary Ellen, Millstone, Natural Brew, Nature's Peak, Pet, Pillsbury, R.W. Knudsen Family, Santa Cruz, Smucker's, White Lily
J.R. Simplot Co.	Culinary Select, Infinity, RoastWorks, Simplot Sweets, Upsides
J&J Snack Foods	Superpretzel, Pretzel Fillers, Pretzelfils, Gourmet Twists, Mr. Twister, Soft Pretzel Bites, Softstix, Soft Pretzel Buns, Hot Knots, Kim & Scott's, Dutch Twist, Texas Twist, Sandwich Twist, Cinnapretzel, Seriously Twisted!, Barq's, Icee, Luigi's, Arctic Blast, Minute Maid Juice Bars and soft frozen lemonade, Shape Ups, Chill, Mama Tish's, Tio Pepe's, Mrs. Goodcookie, Baker's Best, Camden Creek Bakery, Readi-bake, Country Home, Pretzel Cookie, Icee Peak, Slush Puppy, Java Freeze, California Natural, Funnel Cake Factory, Airpopt
JAB/D.E. Master Blenders	Douwe Eberts, Tea Forte, Peet's Coffee & Tea
JBS USA	5 Star Beef, Aspen Ridge Natural Beef, Blue Ribbon Angus, Cedar River Farms, Chef's Exclusive, Clear River Farms, G.F. Swift 1855 Brand, Liberty Bell, Moyer, Packerland, Showcase Premium Ground Beef Swift
John B. Sanfilippo & Son	Fisher Nuts, Orchard Valley Harvest
Kellogg Co.	All-Bran, Apple Jacks, Austin, Bear Naked, Bran Buds, Cinnamon Crunch, Crispix, Cheez-It, Chips Deluxe, Club, Crunchmania, Cocoa Krispies, Complete, Corn Pops, Cracklin' Oat Bran, Crispix, Eggo, E.L. Fudge, Famous Amos, Froot Loops, Frosted Mini-Wheats, Fruit Streamers, Fudge Shoppe, Go-Tarts, Honey Smacks, Just Right, Kashi, Keebler, Kellogg's Krispy, Kellogg's Corn Flakes, Kellogg's Crunch, Kellogg's Frosted Flakes, Kellogg's Raisin Bran, Kellogg's Smorz, Kellogg's Low Fat Granola, Loma Linda, Morningstar Farms, Murray, Natural Touch, Nutri-Grain, Mini-Swirlz, Mueslix, Pops, Pringles, Product 19, Pop-Tarts, Rice Krispies, Right Bites, Sandies, Smart Start,

BIG FOOD	COMMON BRAND NAMES
Kellogg Co. (cont'd.)	Special K, Soft Batch, Stretch Island, Sunshine, Toasted, Town House, Twistables, Vector, Wheatables, Wholesome and Hearty, Worthington, Yogos, Zesta
Keystone Foods	Poultry, beef, fish especially for quick-service restaurants
Kraft Foods Inc. (also owns Mondelez International)	A1 Steak Sauce, Africana (Romania), Air Crisps, Ali Coffee, Back to Nature, Bagel-Fuls, Better Cheddars, Boca Burger, Bonox, Breakstone's, Bull's-Eye Barbecue Sauce, Café HAG, Calumet Baking Powder Company, Cameo (biscuits), Capri Sun (juice drink), Cheesybite, Charada (Peru), Cheez Whiz, Cheezels (Malaysia), Chicken in a Biskit, Chipsmore (Malaysia, Singapore), Claussen (pickles), Clight, Club Social (crackers), Cool Whip (nondairy whipped cream), CornNuts (snack food), Coronita (Peru), Country Time (powdered drink mix), Cracker Barrel Cheese, Crystal Light, Dadák (coffee) (Czech Republic), Dairylea (Europe), Easy Cheese, Eden Cheese (Philippines), El Caserío (Spain), Estrella (Sweden), Field (Peru), Figaro (Chocolate) (Slovakia), Filipinos (snack food) (Spain, Portugal), Fontaneda (biscuits) (Spain), Fudgee-O (Canada), General Foods International, Gevalia (Sweden), Gyõri (biscuits) (Hungary), Grey Poupon (mustard), Handi-Snacks, Harvest Crisps, Honey Maid, Hospitals, In-A-Biskit (Australia), Jacob's (biscuits), Japp (Scandinavia), Jell-O (gelatin dessert), Jet-Puffed Marshmallows, Jiagai (China), Knox (gelatin), Knudsen (dairy) (California), Kong Haakon (Norway), Kolonáda (Czech Republic), Kool-Aid (flavored drink mix), Korona (Ukraine), Kraft BBQ Sauce, Kraft Caramels, Kraft Macaroni and Cheese, Kraft Dinner (Canada), Kraft Easy Mac, Kraft Mayo, Kraft Bagelfuls, Kraft Peanut Butter (Canada), Kraft Singles (pasteurized prepared cheese product), Kraft Sandwich Spread, Kraker Bran, Lacta (Brazil, Greece), Liga (Netherlands), Lucky crackers (Taiwan), Lunchables, Lyuks (potato chips) (Ukraine), Maarud (potato chips) (Norway), Maxwell House (coffee), Mellow Bird's Coffee (United Kingdom), MiO, Miracle Whip (salad dressing spread), Miracoli (Germany), Mostro (Peru), Nabob (coffee) (Canada), Non-Stop (Scandinavia), O'boy (Scandinavia, Estonia), O'smile (Taiwan), Onko (coffee), Opavia (Czech Republic, Slovakia), Orchard Crisps, ORO Saiwa, Oscar Mayer, Grated Parmesan Cheese, Pacific crackers (China), Philadelphia cream cheese, Pigrolac, Planters, Poiana (Romania), Polly-O (cheese), Premium (a Nabisco brand of saltine crackers),

BIG FOOD	COMMON BRAND NAMES
Kraft Foods Inc. (also owns Mondelez International) (cont'd.)	Pretzels, P'tit Québec, Pure Kraft Salad Dressings, Ritz Metro, Royal baking powder, Saiwa (Italian Division of Nabisco), Seven Seas (salad dressings), Saimaza (Spain), Sanka (decaffeinated coffee), Shake'N Bake, Simmenthal (canned meat), Snackabouts, South Beach Living, Starbucks (grocery store items), Stove Top (stuffing), Svoge (Bulgaria), Swiss Crackers, Sugar Wafers, Taco using pods branded as T-Discs), Terrabusi (Kraft Foods Argentina), Tiger Energy Biscuits (Southeast Asia), Toasted Chips, Twisties (Malaysia), Uguan (China), Vegemite (Australia), Velveeta
Lactalis American Group Inc.	President Cheese
Lancaster Colony Corp.	Amish Kitchen, Aunt Vi's, Cardini's, Chatham Village, Girard's, Inn Maid, Jack Daniel's, Mamma Bella, Marshall's, Mary B's, Marzetti, New York Brand, Reames, Romanoff, Sister Schubert's, T. Marzetti, Pfeiffer
Land O'Lakes Inc.	Alpine Lace, Kozy Shack, Land O'Lakes
Leprino Foods Co.	Private label cheese
Maple Leaf Foods	Ben's, Bon Matin, Canada Bread Co., Dempster's, Maple Leaf, Mina, Natural Selections, New York Bakery Co., Olivieri, Prime Turkey, POM, Schneider's, Tenderflake, Vilaggio
Mars Inc.	3 Musketeers, Alterra Coffee Roasters, Altoids, Banfield Pet Hospital, Bright Tea Co., Cesar, Cocoavia, Combos, Doublemint, Dove, Ethel-M, Extra, Flavia, Kudos, M&Ms, Milky Way, Orbit, Pedigree, Royal Canin, Seeds of Change, Sheba, Skittles, Snickers, Starburst, Twix, Uncle Ben's, Waltham, Whiskas, Wisdom Panel
McCain Foods	Brew City, Ellios, McCain, Wong Wing
McCormick & Co. Inc.	McCormick, Zatarain's, Simply Asia, Thai Kitchen, Club House, Golden Dipt, Mojave, Old Bay, Produce Partners
McKee Foods Corp.	Fieldstone Bakery, Heartland, Little Debbie, Sunbelt

BIG FOOD	COMMON BRAND NAMES
Michael Foods	Papetti's, M.G. Waldbaum, Abbotsford, Crystal Farms, Better'n Eggs, Simply Potatoes, AllWhites, Inovatech Egg Products
Miller Coors	Henry Weinhard, Icehouse, Leinenkugel, Mickey's Malt Liquor, Miller Chill, Miller Genuine Draft (international brand), Miller Genuine Draft Light, Miller High Life, Miller Lite, Milwaukee's Best, Milwaukee's Best Ice, Milwaukee's Best Light, Olde English 800 Malt Liquor, Steel Reserve, Southpaw Light, Crispin, Fox Barrell
MOM Brands	Better Oats, Bear River Valley, Farina Mills, Malt-O-Meal, Mom's Best, Sally's, Three Sisters, Naturally Nora, Coco Wheats
Mondelez International (owned by Kraft Foods)	Back to Nature, Barni, Bel Vita, Chips Ahoy, Club Social, Honey Maid, Lu, Nabisco, Newtons, Oreo, Ritz, Triscuit, Tuc, Wheat Thins; Chocolate: Cadbury, Cadbury Dairy Milk, Cote d'Or, Lacta, Milka, Toblerone; Gum and candy: Cadbury, Chiclets, Green & Black's, Halls, Stride, Trident; Grocery: Carte Noir, Jacobs, Kenco, Philadelphia, Tang, Tassimo
National Grape Cooperative	Bama, Welch's
Nestlé (United States and Canada)	Acqua Panna, Aero, After Eight, Alpo, Antica Gelateria del Corso, Aquarel, Arrowhead, Baby Ruth, Baci, Baerenmarke, Beggin' Strips, Belté, Beneful, Boost, Buitoni, Butterfinger, Buxton, Cailler, Calistoga, Carnation, Cat Chow, Cerelac, Cerevita, Chamyto, Cheerios (European license), Chef, Chef-Mate, Chocapic, Cini Minis, Clinutren, Coffee-Mate, Contrex, Cookie Crisp, Dar Natury, Davigel, Davifrais, Deer Park, Delissio, Dibs, Dog Chow, Dreyer's, Edy's Slow Churned, Dibs, Häagen-Dazs, Drumstick, Skinny Cow, Nestlé Toll House, Nestlé Carnation, Nestlé Push-Up, Frosty Paws, Eskimo Pie, Ecco, Estrelitas, EveryDay, Extrême, Fancy Feast, Felix, Fitness, Friskies, Gerber, Gerber Graduates, Good Start, Gourmet, Herta, Hot Pockets, Lean Pockets, Ice Mountain, Impact, Jenny Craig, Juicy Juice, Kit Kat, La Cremeria, La Laitière, Lean Cuisine, Levissima, Lion, Maggi, Maxibon, Milo, Minor's, Mövenpick, Mucilon, NaturNes, Nero, Nescafé, Nescau, Nespresso, Nesquik, Nestea, Nestlé, Nestlé Crunch, One, Optifast, Orion, Peptamen, Perrier, Perugina, Poland Spring, PowerBar, Pro Plan, Pure Life, Purina, Quality Street, Real Dairy, Resource, S.Pellegrino, Smarties, Stouffer's, Sweet Leaf Tea, Taster's Choice, Thomy, Tidy Cats, Toronto, Trio, Tribe Mediterranean Foods, Vittel, Wonka, Yorkie

BIG FOOD	COMMON BRAND NAMES
OSI Group	Amick Farms LLC (Batesburg, SC, and Hurlock, MD), OSI China, OSI Europe, GenOSI Inc. (Philippines), K&K Foods Ltd. (Taiwan), Vista Processed Foods (India), DaOSI (Joint Venture with Doyoo Group, China), OJC (Joint Venture with JC Comsa, China), Fair Oaks Farms LLC (Pleasant Prairie, WI), Nation Pizza and Foods (Schaumburg, IL)
Parmalat Canada	Astro, Balderson, Beatrice, Black Diamond, La Crème, Lactantia, Lactis, Parmalat, Sensational Soy
PepsiCo Inc.	Amp, Aquafina, Aunt Jemima, Baken-Ets, Cap'n Crunch, Cheetos, Chester's, Cracker Jack, Diet Pepsi, Dole (license), Doritos, El Isleno, Ethos, Fiesta, Frappuccino, Flat Earth, Fritos, Funyuns, G2, G Natural, Gamesa, Gatorade, Grandma's Cookies, Hickory Sticks, Hostess Potato Chips, Izze, Kas Mas, King Vitaman, Lay's, Life, Lipton (partnership), Manzanita, Matador, Mirinda, Miss Vickie's, Mother's, Mountain Dew, Mug, Munchies, Muncos, Naked Juice, Near East, No Fear, Nobby Nuts, Ocean Spray (licensed), O'Grady's, Parkers, Pasta Roni, Pepsi, Propel, Quaker, Quisp, Rice-A-Roni, Rold Gold, Ruffles, Sabritas, Sabritones, Santitas, Seattle's Best Coffee, 7UP, Sierra Mist, Slice, Smartfood, Smith's, SoBe, South Beach, Stacy's, Storm, SunChips, Tazo, Tostitos, Tropicana, True North, Walkers
Perdue Farms	Perdue, Hans, Harvestland, Coleman Natural, Draper Valley Farms, Petaluma/Rosie, Rocky
Pilgrim's Pride	EatWellStayHealthy, EggsPlus, Pilgrim's Pride, Easy Entrée, Wing Dings
Pinnacle Foods	Armour, Aunt Jemima, Bernstein's, Birds Eye, Birds Eye C&W, Freshlike, Brooks, Celeste, Comstock Wilderness, Duncan Hines, Greenwood, Hungry-Man, Husman's, Lender's, Log Cabin, McKenzie's, Mrs. Butterworth's, Mrs. Paul's, Nalley, Open Pit, Riviera, Swanson, Snyder of Berlin, Tim's, Van de Kamp's, Vlasic, Voila!
Post Foods (Hearthside Foods)	Alpha-Bits, Golden Crisp, Erewhon, Good Mornings, Grape-Nuts, Great Grains, Honey Bunches of Oats, Honeycomb, New Morning, Pebbles, Post, Post Selects, Spoon Size Shredded Wheat, Waffle Crisp, Golden Temple, Peace Cereal, Willamette Valley Granola

BIG FOOD	COMMON BRAND NAMES
Prairie Farms Dairy Inc.	Belfonte, Coleman Dairy, Hiland Dairy, LuVel, Muller Pinehurst, North Star, Old Recipe, Pevely, Prairie Farms, Southern Belle, Swiss Valley, Tiller Foods, Turner Dairy
Reser's Fine Foods	Reser's, Baja Café, Main St. Bistro, Sidari's, Stonemill Kitchens, American Classics
Rich Products Corp.	Seapack, FarmRich, Carvel, Freal, Byrons BBQ, Casa Meatballs, French Meadow Bakery, Rich's Coffee Rich
Sanderson Farms	Sanderson Farms fresh and frozen poultry
Saputo Inc. (Canada)	Alexis de Portneuf, Armstrong, Baxter, Black Creek, Dairyland, DairyStar, Danscorella, Dragone, DuVillage 1860, Friendship, Frigo, Frigo Cheese Heads, Great Midwest, Hop & Go, King's Choice, Kingsey, La Paulina, Lorraine, Milk2Go, Neilson, Nutrilait, Organic Creamery, Ricrem, Rondeau, Salemville, Saputo, Stella, Treasure Cave, Vachon
Sargento Foods Inc.	Sargento cheese and snacks
Schreiber Foods Inc.	American Heritage, Chuck E. Cheese, Clearfield Deli, Cooper, La Feria, Menu, Pauly, Raskas, Schreiber, School Choice
Schwan Food Co.	Big Daddy's, Edwards, Freschetta, Larry's, LiveSmart, Minh, Mrs. Smith's, Pagoda Express, Red Baron, Schwan's, Tony's
Seaboard Corp.	Seaboard Farms, Prairie Fresh, a Taste like No Other, Daily's, Daily's Premium Meats Since 1893, High Plains Bioenergy, Prairie Fresh Prime, Seaboard Foods, Buffet Brand and Seaboard Farms, Inc.
Seneca Foods Inc.	Seneca, Libby's, Aunt Nellie's Farm Kitchen, Stokely's, Read, Festal
Smithfield Foods, Inc.	Aoste, Armour, Big 8's, Bistro Naturals, Campofrio, Carando, Cook's, Cumberland Gap, Curly's, Del Mare, Dinner Bell, Eckrich, Ember Farms, Esskay, Farmland, Farmstead, First Prize, Great, Gwaltney, Healthy Ones, Hunter, Jamestown, John Morrell, Krakus, Kretschmar, Lunch Maker, Lykes, Margherita, Mosey's, Patrick Cudahy, Patrick's Pride, Paula Deen, Peyton's, Rath, Realean, Rodeo, Smithfield Lean Generation Pork, Smithfield Premium, Sunnyland, the Peanut Shop, Tobin's, Valleydale

BIG FOOD	COMMON BRAND NAMES
Snyder's-Lance Inc.	Snyder's of Hanover, Lance Fresh, Lance Private Brands, Late July, Cape Cod, Krunchers, Tom's, Grande, Archway Cookie, eat smart, Stella D'oro, Jay's, Oke-Doke, Padrino's
Sunkist Growers	Sunkist
TreeHouse Foods Inc.	Farman's, Nalley, Mocha Mix, Peter Piper, Rod's, Second Nature, Steinfeld's, Nature's Goodness, Naturally Fresh, Bennett's, Hoffman House, Roddenberry, Sturm Foods
Tyson Foods, Inc.	Any'tizers, Bonici, Cavanaugh, Chairman's Reserve, Cobb, Colonial, Corn King, Cut & Ready, Delightful Farms, Deli Slices, Doskocil, Golden Trophy, Grilled & Ready, Hot Wings, IBP, Jefferson Meats, Joseph Copperfield's & Sons, Lady Aster, Mexican Original, Mr. Nuccio, Open Prairie Natural Angus, Original Wraps Our American Favorite, Pizza Topper, Pizzano, Readi Rise, Reuben, Russer, Solo Serves, Star Ranch Angus, Supreme Tender, Tastybird, Tenderpress, Thorn Apple Valley, Trimmed & Ready, Tyson, Weaver, Wilson, Wilson Foodservice, Wright, Wunderbar
Unilever North America	Amora, Becel, Ben & Jerry's, Bertolli, Blue Band, Breyers, Calve, CarbSmart, Carte d'Or, Cornetto, Country Crock, Doriana, Flora, Good Humor, Heart/Heartbrand, Hellmann's, Knorr, Lipton, Magnum, Promise, Rama, Shedd's, Slim-Fast, Solero
Wells Enterprises Inc.	Blue Bunny, Bomb Pops, 2nd St. Creamery, Weight Watchers (licensed), Yoplait (licensed)
Weston Foods	Arnold, Country Harvest, D'Italiano, Entenmann's, Freihofer's, Neilson, Stroehmann, Thomas', Weston, Wonder
WhiteWave Foods	Alpro, Horizon Organic, International Delight, Silk

(From foodprocessing.com and the Cornucopia Institute)

Common Food Brands and Recommended Alternatives

Some of the products listed are my ideal, while others are simply better alternatives. You have to decide what is best for you. Some brands come from companies that are doing everything, or almost everything, "right" when sourcing ingredients, processing, and marketing the product to you, and some are not. But I can assure you that even the worst on my list could very well be better than what you are currently doing, so anything is a step in the right direction as far as I am concerned.

I modeled this guide after one of my local monstrous markets, aisle by aisle. And I tried not to be too biased here, sticking with items available in many mainstream food stores today. Note that you may be able to find *decent, cost-effective* versions of the items listed at Whole Foods Market under their exclusive 365 Everyday Value brand.

You decide what works best for you. By the way, I am sure that I missed some really good buys, as the food marketplace is forever changing, so surely stay updated and informed by following me on Facebook: StefanieSacks; Twitter: @Stefanie_Sacks; or by tuning in to my weekly *Stirring the Pot* radio show, which you can catch by signing up for my weekly blog at stefaniesacks.com. I will always have something to offer about good food brands.

THE EDGE OF THE MARKETPLACE

COMMON FOODS (in no specific order)	RECOMMENDED ALTERNATIVES
REFRIGERATED	
Dairy and Eggs	
Milk	Natural by Nature, Organic Valley, Woodstock, Ronnybrook
Nondairy milks	Rice Dream, Silk, So Delicious, Zen
Creamers (dairy and nondairy)	Blue Diamond, Organic Valley, Silk, So Delicious
Whipped cream	Natural by Nature
Cheese (blocks, shreds, slices, sticks)	Organic Valley
Processed cheese food	Organic Valley
Cream cheese, sour cream, cottage cheese, ricotta cheese	Natural by Nature, Organic Valley
Yogurt (dairy and nondairy)	Almond Dream, Brown Cow, Chobani, Fage, Green Valley Organics, Maple Hill Creamery, Ricera, Seven Stars, Siggi's, Silk, So Delicious, Trimona, Wallaby, Whole Soy
Yogurt drinks	Lifeway, Ronnybrook, Siggi's
Yogurt tubes	Siggi's

COMMON FOODS (in no specific order)	RECOMMENDED ALTERNATIVES
Pudding (dairy and nondairy)	Kozy Shack, Zen
Butter	Cabot, Kate's, Land O'Lakes, Natural by Nature, Organic Valley, Stonyfield, Woodstock
Margarine	Earth Balance, Spectrum Spread
Egg substitute	Eggology, Organic Valley Egg Whites
Juice and Other Beverages	
Orange/grapefruit juice	Simply Beverages
Lemonade/limeade	Simply Beverages
Iced tea	Newman's Own
Lunch Meats	
Deli meats	Applegate Farms, Wellshire Farms
Bacon, sausage, jerky	Applegate Farms, Garrett County, Shelton's
Hot dogs	Applegate Farms, Garrett County, Wellshire Farms
Other	
Dough (cookies, biscuits, crusts)	Immaculate Baking Company

COMMON FOODS (in no specific order)	RECOMMENDED ALTERNATIVES
Hummus	Abraham's, Cedar's Natural Select, Tribe
Pickles	Bubbies, Real Pickles

FROZEN	

Produce	
Vegetables	Birds Eye, Cascadian Farms, Earthbound Farms, Green Giant, Woodstock Farms
Fruit	Cascadian Farms, Dole, Woodstock Farms, Wyman's,
Potatoes	Alexia, Cascadian Farms

Prepared Foods	
Meals	Amy's, Bombay Kitchen, Cedarlane Natural Foods, Ethnic Gourmet, LYFE Kitchen, Moosewood, Seeds of Change
Pizza	American Flatbread, Amy's, Moosewood Organic Classics, Udi's
Veggie burgers	Dr. Praeger's, Garden, Harvest, Sunshine
Dumplings	Ling Ling
Pierogies	Mrs. T's

COMMON FOODS (in no specific order)	RECOMMENDED ALTERNATIVES
Breakfast Foods/Bakery	
Waffles	Earth's Best, LifeStream, Van's
Muffins	Kinnikinnick, Udi's, Vitalicious
Breads, bagels, "English" muffins, tortillas	Alvarado St. Bakery, Berlin Bakery, Canyon Bakehouse, Ezekiel, Food for Life, Garden of Eatin', Glutino, Manna, Rudi's, Shiloh Farms, Udi's
Blintzes	Ian's
Doughnuts and other baked goods	Foods by George, Kinnikinnick
Meats, Poultry, and Fish	
Sausage	Applegate Farms, Shelton's
Burgers	Coleman Natural Beef Burger, Shelton's Turkey Burgers
Chicken nuggets, tenders, and patties	Applegate Farms, Bell & Evans, Dr. Praeger's, Ian's
Fish sticks and patties	Dr. Praeger's, Ecofish, Ian's, Natural Sea
Sweets	
Cool whipiness	Truwhip

COMMON FOODS (in no specific order)	RECOMMENDED ALTERNATIVES
Ice cream, frozen yogurt, and sorbet (dairy and nondairy)	Ben & Jerry's, Breyer's Organic, Ciao Bella, Julie's, Rice Dream, Ronnybrook, Sharon's, So Delicious, Steve's, Stonyfield Farms
Ice pops	Cascadian Farms (juice), Ciao Bella, Cool Fruits Fruit Juice Squeezers, Edy's (real fruit bars), Just Pikt (juice), Smooze
Cookies	French Meadow Bakery, Immaculate Baking Company
MEAT, POULTRY, PORK, AND FISH	
Beef and pork	USDA organic and/or look for labels bearing the Animal Welfare Approved or Certified Humane label. If you want meats with the highest welfare standards, visit animalwelfareapproved.org or certifiedhumane.org to find farmers with this certification (you can order items online)
Poultry	USDA organic and/or look for labels bearing the Animal Welfare Approved or Certified Humane label; if you can't find any, check out Bell & Evans, Eberly's, D'Artagnan, Free Bird, Murray's; and of course feel free to order online as noted above
Fish	Go to your local fishmonger; always ask questions at the counter using the Monterey Bay Aquarium Seafood Watch as your guide

THE INNARDS OF THE MARKETPLACE

COMMON FOODS	THEIR BETTER HALVES
BEVERAGES	
Juice	Apple & Eve (organic), Honest, Knudsen, Newman's, Santa Cruz
Soda	Blue Sky, Flavored Pellegrino or Poland GuS, Izze, Knudsen, Reed's, Santa Cruz, Spring seltzer
Sports drinks	Emergen-C electrolyte powder, Harvest Bay coconut water or other unflavored option, Titan Tea
Iced tea	Honest, Ito En, Teas' Tea, Titan Tea
Tea and coffee	Celestial Seasonings, Tazo, Traditional Medicinals, Twinings
Hot chocolate (and chocolate syrup)	Ah!laska, Green & Blacks
BREADS	
Bread	Canyon Bakehouse, Matthew's, the Baker, Rudi's, Udi's, Vermont Bread Co.
Pita	Garden of Eatin' Bible Bread
"English" muffins	Matthew's, Rudi's, Vermont Baking Co.
Bread crumbs and panko	Glutino, Ian's, Jaclyn's, Schar

COMMON FOODS	THEIR BETTER HALVES
Croutons	Edward & Sons, Fresh Gourmet
CRACKERS, COOKIES, AND BOXED BAKERY	
Crackers	
Flaky round crackers	Barbara's Rite Rounds Lite, Late July
Cheese crackers	Barbara's Cheese Bites, Back to Nature Crispy Cheddars, Late July Bite Size Cheddar Cheese
"Fish" crackers	Annie's Naturals Cheddar Bunnies, Good Health Gold Fish, Our Family Farm Captain's Catch Baked Cheese Crackers, Pepperidge Farm
Salty crackers (oyster, too)	Barbara's Wheatines, Hain Oyster Crackers, Suzie's Salted Crackers
Woven wheat crackers	Barbara's Wheatines, Back to Nature Harvest Whole Wheat
Thin wheat crackers	Hain Wheatettes
Rice cakes/crackers	Edward & Sons, Lundberg, Quaker (plain), San-J, Sesmark
Other crackers	Absolutely Gluten Free, Ak-Mak, Blue Diamond Nut Thins, Glutino, Mary's Gone
Cookies and Boxed Bakery	
Chocolate chip cookies	Back to Nature, Brent & Sam's, Newman's Own, Pamela's

COMMON FOODS	THEIR BETTER HALVES
Sandwich cream cookies	Back to Nature, Glutino, Newman-O's
Oatmeal cookies	Back to Nature, Newman's Own Hermits
Graham crackers	Annie's Naturals, Barbara's Go Go Grahams, Hain, Mi-Del, New Morning
Animal crackers	Annie's Naturals, Barbara's Snackimals, Hain
Fig bars	Barbara's Fig Bars, Fig Newmans
Other cookies	Back to Nature, Bahlsen Jules Destrooper, Enjoy Life Foods, Loacker Quadratini, Mary's Gone, Mi-Del, Pamela's
Granola bars	Bliss Bar, Health Valley Granola Bars
"Energy" bars	Bliss, Bumble, Greens, Kind, Luna, Oskri
CHIPS AND OTHER CRUNCH	
Popcorn (bagged)	Bearitos, Boston Lite, Popcorn Indiana
Popcorn (microwave)	Bearitos, Newman's Own, Quinn Popcorn
Caramel corn	Popcorn Indiana
Tortilla chips	Bearitos, Garden of Eatin', Green Mountain Gringo, Kettle, Xochitl
Flavored tortilla chips	Garden of Eatin', Late July

COMMON FOODS	THEIR BETTER HALVES
Cheesy puffs	Bearitos Cheddar Puffs, Little Bear Crunchitos, Robert's American (Pirate Booty, Tings)
Potato chips	Kettle Brand, Michael Season's, Terra
Vegetable chips	Terra
Pretzels	Glutino, Newman's Own, Snyder's
PASTA, SAUCE, CANNED GOODS, AND PREPARED MEALS	
Pasta and Sauce	
Pasta	Ancient Harvest, Barilla, Bionaturae, DeBoles, DeCecco, Eden, Hodgson Mills, Lundberg, Ronzoni, Sam Mills, Tinkyada
Pasta and pizza sauce	Amy's, Bionaturae, Cucina Antica, Emeril's, Lidia's, Muir Glen, Newman's Own, Rao's, Seeds of Change, Victoria, Walnut Acres
Tomato sauce	Colavita, Contadina, Hunt's, Muir Glen, Pomi, Red Pack
Canned Goods and Prepared Meals	
Canned vegetables	Del Monte (select items), Field Day, Green Giant (select items)
Canned seafood	Crown Prince, Deep Sea, Natural Sea, Wild Catch
Pasta with meat	Annie's Naturals Ravioli

COMMON FOODS	THEIR BETTER HALVES
Macaroni and cheese	Annie's Naturals, Back to Nature
Meal helper packs	Fantastic, Mrs. Leeper's, Simply Organic
Meal seasoning packs and gravies	Bearitos, Hain, Simply Organic
SOUPS, SALAD, PICKLED PICKIN'S, AND CONDIMENTS	
Soups	Amy's, Health Valley, Muir Glen, Shari Ann's, Shelton's, Walnut Acres, Wolfgang Puck
Broth	Emeril's, Health Valley, Imagine, Kitchen Basics, Organic Gourmet, Pacific
Bouillon	Better Than Bouillon, Organic Gourmet, Rapunzel
Salsa	Amy's, Desert Pepper Trading Company, Enrico's, Frontera, Green Mountain Gringo, Muir Glen, Newman's Own
Salad dressing	Annie's Naturals, Newman's Own, Organicville, Seeds of Change, Simply Organic (dry mix), Spectrum, Stonewall Kitchen
Oils	Eden, Hain, Spectrum
Vinegars	Hain, Spectrum
Pickles	Back to Nature, Bubbies, McClure's, Rick's Picks, Woodstock

COMMON FOODS	THEIR BETTER HALVES
Olives, capers, peppers, sun-dried tomatoes, hearts of palm	Mediterranean Organic, Native Forest
Mustard	Grey Poupon, Gulden's, Organicville, Westbrae Natural
Ketchup	Annie's Naturals, Muir Glen, Organicville, Westbrae Natural
Mayonnaise	Hain, Nasoya, Spectrum Naturals, Woodstock
Soy sauce/Tamari	Eden, San-J
Mirin	Eden
Teriyaki (and other Asian-influenced sauces)	San-J, Thai Kitchen, Veri Veri
Steak sauce	Annie's Naturals, Newman's Own
Barbecue sauce	Annie's Naturals, Organicville
Hot sauce	Arizona's Peppers, Melinda's, Organicville
Worcestershire sauce	The Wizards
BAKING, SWEETS, SUGAR, AND SPICE	
Flours	Arrowhead Mills, Bob's Red Mill, Hodgson Mills
Baking mixes	Bob's Red Mill, Cherrybrook Kitchen, Dr. Oetker (some products), Pamela's

COMMON FOODS	THEIR BETTER HALVES
Food colorings	India Tree
Sprinkles and decorations	India Tree, Let's Do Organic
Extracts	Frontier, Simply Organic
Chocolate chips	Chocolate Dream, Enjoy Life Foods, Ghiradelli, Sunspire
Gelatin desserts	Simply Delish
Ice cream cones	Let's Do Organic
Sugar	Domino, Florida Crystals, Hain, Wholesome Sweeteners, Woodstock
Maple syrup (the real stuff)	Maple Grove Farms, Shady Maple Farms, Springtree; any 100 percent pure maple syrup
Other real sweeteners	Eden, Lundberg, Wholesome Sweeteners
Spices	Frontier, Simply Organic
CEREAL AND OTHER "BREAKFAST" ITEMS	
Cheerio-like cereals	Barbara's Apple Cinnamon O's, Barbara's Breakfast O's, Cascadian Farms Purely O's, Cheerios (plain if you must), Kashi Heart to Heart, New Morning Apple Cinnamon Oatios, New Morning Honey Almond Oatios; New Morning Oatios

COMMON FOODS	THEIR BETTER HALVES
Chex-like cereals	Cascadian Farms Multigrain Squares, Health Valley Rice Crunch-Ems, Nature's Path Heritage Bites
Cocoa crispiness	EnviroKidz Koala Crisps, New Morning Cocoa Crispy Rice, New Morning Cocomotion
Corn flakiness	Arrowhead Mills Spelt, Kamut, or Amaranth Flakes; Barbara's Corn Flakes; Erewhon Corn Flakes; Nature's Path Corn Flakes; Kashi Whole Grain Flakes;
Frosted flakiness	Arrowhead Mills Organic Oat Bran Flakes
Fruit loopiness	Barbara's Fruity Punch, New Morning Fruit-E-O's
Raisin braniness	Cascadian Farms, Erewhon, Health Valley Raisin Bran
Rice crispiness	Erewhon Crispy Brown Rice, Kellogg's Rice Krispies (plain if you must)
Shredded wheatiness	Arrowhead Mills Shredded Wheat (unsweetened and sweetened), Barbara's Shredded Spoonfuls, Barbara's Shredded Wheat, Kashi Autumn Wheat
Combs of honey	EnviroKidz Cheetah Chomps
Captain crunchiness	Barbara's Peanut Butter Puffins, EnviroKidz Peanut Butter Panda Puffs

COMMON FOODS	THEIR BETTER HALVES
Granola	Back to Nature Granola, Baker's Granola and Muesli, Bear Naked Granola, Breadshop, Galaxy Granola, Health Valley Granola, Udi's
Oatmeal (rolled oats)	Bob's Red Mill rolled oats
Muesli	Alpen, Familia
Packages of oatmealiness (with added sugar)	Arrowhead Mills, Country Choice, Erewhon, Kashi, Nature's Path, Quaker, Uncle Sam's Oatmeal
Cereal in a bar	Barbara's, Health Valley, Kashi, Nature's Choice, Nature's Path
Pancake/waffle mix	Arrowhead Mills, Bob's Red Mill, Maple Grove Farms, Pamela's
Fruit-filled toaster tarts	Amy's Toaster Pops, Health Valley Tarts
FRUITY AND NUTTY SNACKS	
Applesauce	Eden, Santa Cruz, Vermont Organic, Mott's (without added sugar)
Jam and preserves	Bionature Fruit Spreads, Bon Maman Cascadian, Farms, Harvest Moon, Polaner
Canned fruit	Native Forest
Dried fruit	Earthbound Farms, Peeled, Sunmaid (select varieties), Tree of Life, Woodstock

COMMON FOODS	THEIR BETTER HALVES
Bars	Bumble, Health Warrior Chia Bars, Kate's Real Food Bars, Kind Bars, Oskri, The Pure Bar
Fruit leather	Matt's Munchies, Stretch Island
Fruit snacks	Annie's Naturals Gummy Bunnies
Nut butters (peanut, almond, cashew, etc.)	Arrowhead Mills, MaraNatha, Peanut Butter & Co., Smucker's Naturals, Tree of Life, Woodstock
CANDY (CHECK OUT NATURALCANDYSTORE.COM)	
Gummy candies	Surf Sweets, Yummy Earth
Jelly beans	Surf Sweets
Licorice	Candy Tree, Newman's Own, Panda
Lollipops	Candy Tree, Yummy Earth
Bubble gum	Glee Gum, Tree Hugger
Chocolate	Green & Black's, Lake Champlain, Lundt, Newman's Own, Rapunzel, Tropical Source, Valrhona, Vivani
Colored chocolate candies	Sunspire, Unreal
Peanut butter cups	Justin's, Newman's Own, Unreal

COMMON FOODS	THEIR BETTER HALVES
Chocolate, nutty bars	Justin's, Unreal
Gum	Glee Gum
Mints	VerMints
BABY FOOD	
Formula	Baby's Only Organic (though surely speak to your doctor about your baby and formula), Earth's Best
Staged purées	Earth's Best, Ella's Kitchen,Gerber Organic, Happy Baby, Plum Organics
Puffs and other snacks	Happy Puffs, Healthy Times teething biscuits
INTERNATIONAL	
Asian noodles and noodle soups	Annie Chun's
Asian seasoning sauces	Eden, San-J, Veri Veri
Coconut milk	Native Forest, Thai Kitchen
Chili pastes and spice rubs	Thai Kitchen
Taco kits (and shells)	Bearitos
Refried beans and other Tex-Mex add-ons	Amy's, Bearitos

COMMON FOODS	THEIR BETTER HALVES
RICE AND BEANS	
Canned (and boxed) beans	Eden, Goya (select), Westbrae Natural
Seasoned beans	Amy's, Eden, Natural, Shari Ann's, Walnut Acres, Westbrae
Rice	Lundberg, Rice Select
Rice mixes	Casbah, Lundberg, Near East, Rice Select

Keeping It Fresh, Warding Off Waste

The following are some storage tips that should offer a little direction for keeping your food as fresh and safe as it can be.

BASIC TIPS
- Use glass storage containers.
- Buy products that boast BPA-free packaging.
- Follow the two-hour rule (all foods needing refrigeration or freezing can typically be left out at a cool room temperature for *only two hours*).
- If defrosting, do so in the fridge.
- Keep foods tightly covered in and out of the fridge or freezer.
- Always check storage directions on food labels.
- Foods typically stay fresher if kept in the fridge or freezer.
- For information on composting, check out makedirtnotwaste.org.

YOUR PANTRY

For more specific information, check out eatbydate.com.

DRIED HERBS AND SPICES
- Ground spices last six months to one year stored in a cool, dry place once opened.
- Whole spices last two to three years in a cool, dry place once opened.
- Herbs last six months to one year in a cool, dry place.

OILS
- All oils, once opened, should be stored in the fridge; otherwise they will go rancid quickly. If kept cool, they can last for up to one year.
- Though for olive oil, store in a cool, dark place; if you store it in the fridge, it will solidify. Once opened, olive oil can last for up to six months.

- As each type of oil has its own shelf life, you really have to follow your nose here. Most oils, if stored properly, last for up to one year. But do note that almond oil and walnut oil most readily go rancid, so buy them in small quantities, store them in the fridge, and use them quickly.

VINEGARS
- Store unopened in a cool, dark place, tightly capped, for two years. Once opened, vinegar is most likely good for six months to a year

CONDIMENTS AND SAUCES (SWEETENERS, TOO)
- Unopened in the pantry, condiments and sauces can last up to one year (or even longer).
- Once opened, if stored tightly capped in the fridge, condiments can last for up to six months; soy sauce can last for a year.
- Always store opened sauces and condiments in the fridge, including mustard, ketchup, mayonnaise, and even maple syrup.
- Other liquid sweeteners can be stored in a cool, dark place for up to one year.

CANNED GOODS (BOTTLES AND BOXES, TOO)
- Store unopened in a cool, dry place; once opened, move it to the fridge (if perishable), making sure lids are tightly secured.
- Whatever the good, each has its own shelf life. Let your sight, smell, and taste guide you once you open it. Vegetables, broths, soups, or brews as well as anything meat will keep for three days to one week; jarred fruits, jams, and nut butters will keep for roughly three months, sometimes a little longer.

PASTA, GRAINS, AND DRIED BEANS
- Pasta, if kept dry and in an airtight container, can last for years; check package for details.
- Store whole grains in a closed bag or airtight container in a cool, dry place for three to four months, in the fridge for up to six months, or in the freezer for up to a year.
- Store milled grains (flour) in the fridge or freezer for up to six months.
- Dried beans will keep for one year; colder temperatures increase shelf life.
- Canned beans will keep for three years.

BREADS, BAKERY, AND CEREAL
- A typical loaf will last roughly five to seven days out of the fridge, but if kept cool it can last one to two weeks.

- Fresh-baked breads last one to two days at room temperature. You can move to the fridge after that to keep for up to a week and heat in toaster oven to soften before consumption.
- Breads that come from the freezer, like really grainy and sprouted breads, should be kept in the freezer or fridge at all times. In the freezer they can last for up to three months; in the fridge, they will keep for one to two weeks.
- Highly processed cereals, once opened, can last in a cool, dark place for three to four months; less processed ones such as a fresh granola should be kept in the fridge for up to four to six months.

NUTS AND SEEDS
- Once opened, store in the fridge or freezer for six to eight months.

SNACKS
- These can literally last a lifetime if unopened and in your pantry (think Twinkies).
- If opened, most snacks can last a few weeks in the pantry and longer in the fridge.

BAKING
- Anything baking-related (other than yeast and baking powder and soda) can last years unopened in your pantry.
- If opened, keep for a year at best.

FRIDGE AND FREEZER

PRODUCE (FRUITS, VEGETABLES, AND HERBS)
- In the fridge, fruits can last up to one week (sometimes longer); apples and citrus typically last three weeks.
- In the fridge, vegetables last for up to one week. Onions, garlic, winter squash, roots (carrots), and tubers (yams) typically last longer (three weeks).
- Fresh herbs last for up to one week in the fridge; store them in a wet dish towel or paper towel.
- In the freezer, fruits and vegetables can last for up to one year.

MEATS, POULTRY, AND FISH
- Meats, poultry, and fish will keep for one to two days in the fridge or three to four months in the freezer.

DAIRY (MILK, BUTTER, CHEESE, YOGURT, OTHER) AND EGGS
- For milk, always see the expiration date but also use your nose as a guide.
- Butter will keep in the fridge for one month or in the freezer for one year; if opened, it lasts for two weeks.

- Cheeses will keep for various times, depending on the type of cheese; typically softer cheeses will keep for a few weeks, and harder cheese will keep for a few months.
- Eggs will keep for up to thirty days in the fridge.

PREPARED FOODS/LEFTOVERS
- Prepared foods and leftovers will keep for three to four days in the fridge or three to six months in the freezer.

BREADS AND BAKERY
- Breads and baked goods will keep for two to three days at room temperature (unless filled with chemical preservatives), one to two weeks in the fridge or three to six months in the freezer.

SWEET TREATS
- Ice creams, pops, and desserts will typically last for six months to one year, though watch out for freezer burn.

The Practical Whole Foods Pantry

Let this shopping list (or parts of it) be your new blueprint for a better relationship with food. Many ingredients within are reflected in the recipes in *What the Fork*.

NONPERISHABLES		PERISHABLES	
GRAINS (whole and other)	CONDIMENTS	VEGETABLES	FRUITS
Amaranth	Tamari—reduced sodium	Asparagus	Lemons/limes
Brown rice	Mirin (or cooking wine)	Avocado	Blueberries/juice
Specialty rice (wild, red, black)	Curry paste	Brussels sprouts	Plums
Quinoa	Roasted red chili paste	Cauliflower	Apples
Oats—steel cut, rolled	Dijon mustard	Celery	Kiwis
Millet	Rice vinegar	Fennel	Grapefruit
Kasha (buckwheat)	Balsamic vinegar	Green beans	Oranges

NONPERISHABLES		PERISHABLES	
Spelt (faro)	Wine vinegar	Peppers	Strawberries
Whole-wheat flour	Cider vinegar	Snap peas	Cantaloupe
Oat flour	Broth (vegetable or chicken)	Winter squash	Pomegranates/juice
Brown rice flour	Coconut milk	Zucchini	Papayas (organic)
Buckwheat flour	Honey	Yams/sweet potatoes	Peaches
Cornmeal (organic)	Brown rice syrup	Carrots	Nectarines
Noodles, Pasta (Rice and Other)	Maple syrup (grade B)	Parsnips	Apricots
100 percent sprouted-grain breads (or other grain breads)	**OILS**	Beets	**PROTEINS**
Tortillas (organic corn, sprouted, other)	Extra virgin olive oil (first cold pressed)	Kale	Tofu
BEANS (CANNED OR DRIED)	Grapeseed oil	Swiss chard	Tempeh
Garbanzos	Sesame oil (light and toasted)	Collard greens	Eggs
Pinto beans	Safflower or sunflower oil	Spinach	Seafood

NONPERISHABLES		PERISHABLES	
Kidney beans	Coconut oil	Broccoli	Canned wild salmon, sardines
Cannellini beans	Walnut oil	Mustard greens	Poultry
Adzuki beans	Flax oil	Bok choy	Pork
Black beans	**DRIED HERBS/ SPICES**	Arugula	Meats
Green lentils	Cinnamon (whole & ground)	Cucumber	**DAIRY AND NONDAIRY**
Red lentils	Cardamom (whole or ground)	Tomatoes/grape tomatoes	Organic milk
Split peas	Cumin	Dandelion greens	Organic cheese (or without hormones and antibiotics)
Split mung beans	Coriander	Watercress	Plain yogurt/kefir
NUTS AND SEEDS	Turmeric	Leaf lettuce	Soy milk (unsweetened)
Almonds	Paprika	Garlic	Oat milk
Walnuts	Chili powder	Ginger	Almond milk
Pecans	Curry powder	Onions	Hazelnut milk
Pine nuts	Garam masala	Scallions	Coconut milk
Cashews	Basil	Leeks	Hempseed milk

NONPERISHABLES		PERISHABLES	
Hazelnuts	Oregano	Shallots	Soy/coconut yogurt
Brazil nuts	Dill	Rosemary	Rice milk
Pumpkin seeds	Cayenne pepper	Thyme	Coconut water
Sunflower seeds	Cloves	Basil	
Flax/flax meal	Non-aluminum baking powder and soda	Sage	
Sesame seeds	Pure vanilla extract	Cilantro	
Black sesame seeds	**GROCERY, OTHER**	Oregano	
Almond butter	Apple juice (organic)	Flat-leaf parsley	
Peanut butter (organic)	Salsa	Mint	
Cashew butter	Unsweetened coconut	Dill	
Tahini (sesame seed butter)	Dark chocolate (70%+)	Local sustainable sea vegetables (if you fancy) such as those from Ocean Approved or Maine Coast sea vegetables	

Redeemable Resources

I consider each and every one of these organizations, efforts, and people the *real-deal* change agents. They are *all* my go-to for everything food, nutrition, health, culinary, and community and a great starting point for you to learn more if you want.

FOOD POLICY, SAFETY, AND ACCOUNTABILITY

Animal Welfare Approved (animalwelfareapproved.org)
Blue Ocean Institute (blueocean.org)
Campaign for a Commercial-Free Childhood (commercialfreechildhood.org)
Center for Food Safety (centerforfoodsafety.org)
Center for Science in the Public Interest (cspi.net)
Consumers Union (consumersunion.org)
Cornucopia Institute (cornucopia.org)
Corporate Accountability International (stopcorporateabuse.org)
Environmental Working Group (ewg.org)
Feeding the 5000 (feeding5k.org)
Food and Water Watch (foodandwaterwatch.org)
Food Day (food day.org)
Food Democracy Now (fooddemocracynow.org)
Food MythBusters (foodmyths.org)
Food Tank (foodtank.org)
GRACE Communications Foundation (gracelinks.org)
Institute for Responsible Technology (responsibletechnology.org)
Just Label It (justlabelit.org)
Monterey Bay Aquarium Seafood Watch (seafoodwatch.org)
Natural Resources Defense Council (nrdc.org)
National Sustainable Agriculture Coalition (sustainableagriculture.net)

Non-GMO Project (nongmoproject.org)
Organic Consumers Association (organicconsumers.org)
A Place at the Table (takepart.com/placeatthetable)
Small Planet Fund (smallplanetfund.org)
Sustainable Table (sustainabletable.org)
Think Eat Save (thinkeatsave.org)
Union of Concerned Scientists (ucsusa.org)
Why Hunger (whyhunger.org)

NUTRITION AND HEALTH

Alliance for Natural Health USA (anh-usa.org)
Center for Mind-Body Medicine (cmbm.org)
Center for Nutrition Advocacy (nutritionadvocacy.org)
Environmental Nutrition (environmentalnutrition.com)
Food Revolution Network (foodrevolution.org)
Institute for Functional Medicine (functionalmedicine.org)
Meatless Monday (meatlessmonday.com)
Monday Campaigns (mondaycampaigns.org)
Tufts Health and Nutrition Letter (tuftshealthletter.com)

CULINARY AND COMMUNITY

Ceres Community Project (ceresproject.org)
Dock to Dish (docktodish.com)
Eat Wild (eatwild.com)
Edible Communities (ediblecommunities.com)
International Association of Culinary Professionals (iacp.com)
James Beard Foundation (jamesbeard.org)
Just Food (justfood.org)
Local Catch (localcatch.org)
Local Harvest (localharvest.org)
Locavores (locavores.com)
Natural Gourmet Institute (naturalgourmetinstitute.com)
Nourish: Food + Community (nourishlife.org)
Slow Food (slowfood.org)
Superfood Drive (superfooddrive.org)
Sustainable Table (sustainabletable.org)
Wholesome Wave (wholesomewave.org)

SCHOOL AND COMMUNITY

Edible Schoolyard (edibleschoolyard.org)
Food Corps (foodcorps.org)
Food Revolution (jamiesfoodrevolution.com)
Ground up Campaign (birdsnestfoundation.com)
Lunch Lessons (lunchlessons.org)
School Food Revolution (jamieoliver.com)
School Garden Curriculum (growtolearn.com)
Veggication (veggication.com)
Wellness in the Schools (wellnessintheschools.org)

SMARTPHONE APPS FOR APPETITES

Dirty Dozen™ (ewg.org)
Eat Local (nrdc.org)
Farmstand (farmstandapp.com)
Food Database™ (ewg.org)
Feedfeed (feedfeed.info)
Food Labels Exposed (animalwelfareapproved.org)
Fooducate (fooducate.com)
Harvest (harvest-app.com)
Non-GMO Project Shopping Guide (nongmoproject.org)
Seafood Watch (montereybayaquarium.org)
True Food (centerforfoodsafety.org)
What's on My Food (whatsonmyfood.org)

FOOD IN THE MEDIA

MUST-SEE MOVIES

American Meat
Betting the Farm
Dirt: the Movie
Fat, Sick & Nearly Dead
Food Fight
Food Inc.
Food Stamped: a Film for Our Times
Forks over Knives

Fresh
The Garden
Genetic Roulette
GMO OMG
Killer at Large
King Corn
A Place at the Table
The Real Dirt on Farmer John
Super Size Me

TED TALKS

Creativity in Cooking Can Solve Our Biggest Challenges (Jose Andrews)

Effects of a High Meat Diet on Public Health (Bob Lawrence)

Factory Farms, Antibiotics and Superbugs (Dr. Lance Price)

Food + Justice = Democracy (LaDonna Redman)

From New York to Africa: Why Food Is Saving the World (Brian Halweil)

A Garden in My Apartment (Britta Riley)

The Global Food Waste Scandal (Tristram Stuart)

The Global Water Footprint of Humanity (Angela Morelli)

Great Tomatoes for All (Michel Nischan)

Green Bronx Machine (Stephen Ritz)

A Guerilla Gardener in South Central LA (Ron Finley)

How Big Business Had the Right Idea but Went Wrong (Andrew Gunther)

How Food Shapes Our Cities (Carolyn Steel)

How I Did Less and Ate Better (Tama Matsuoko Wong)

How I Fell in Love with a Fish (Dan Barber)

The Hungry Farmer—My Moment of Great Disruption (Roger Thurow)

Lunch Lessons (Ann Cooper)

Marketing Food to Children (Anna Lappé)

The Measure of All Things (Fred Kaufman)

Meatless Monday: How a Simple Idea Sparks a Global Health Movement (Peggy Neu)

Obesity + Hunger = 1 Global Food Issue (Ellen Gustafson)

Raising Pigs & Problems (David Wallinga)

Recirculating Farms: Building a Healthy Sustainable Food Culture (Marianne Cufone)

A Subversive Plot (Roger Doiron)

Teach Every Child about Food (Jamie Oliver)

Thinking about Soil (Joel Salatin)

Turning the Farm Bill into the Food Bill (Ken Cook)
A Vision for Sustainable Restaurants (Arthur Potts Dawson)
What's Wrong with Our Food System (Burke Baehr)
What's Wrong with What We Eat (Mark Bittman)
Who Pays the Farm Bill (Wenonah Hauter)
Why I'm a Weekday Vegetarian (Graham Hill)

Acknowledgments

My love for food and cooking began at age three. My parents bought me a wooden play kitchen and when my grandma Lorraine visited, we played restaurant—each time I meticulously prepared her a tuna sandwich on white bread with a pickle while she patiently waited. I guess you can say that I have always had a love for the culinary arts.

To Kathryn Nadeau for letting me into your Naturally Good haven in the 1980s, where I was given the support and freedom to flourish and find my true calling. And to all my food, nutrition, and health goddesses and gods for your passion, inspiration, education, and devotion to changing the way we think about food—you have all been with me through my personal and professional journey. I feel honored to have been touched by all of you whether personally or virtually—Annemarie Colbin, PhD; Mollie Katzen; Dr. Sherry Rogers; Dr. Andrew Weil; Frances Moore Lappé; Mary Cleaver; Michel Nischan; Dr. Tieraona Low Dog; Isobel Contento, PhD, MA; Lora Sporny, EdD, MEd, MA, RDN; Larry Kushi, ScD; Toni Liquori, EdD, MPH; Joan Gussow, EdD, MEd; Randi Wolf, MPH, PhD; Walter Willet, MD, Dr. PH; Fredi Kronenberg, PhD; Ann Cooper; Marion Nestle, PhD, MPH; Lisa Young, PhD, RD, CDN; Mary Beth Augustine, MS, RDN, CDN; Kathie Swift, MS, RDN, LDN; Dr. Stephen Cowan; Scott Berliner, RPH; Rebecca Katz, MS; Julie Negrin, MS, CN; Ellie Krieger, MS, RDN; and John Bagnulo, MPH, RDN, PhD.

Stephen Weiss, your imprint in life and death will be with me forever. Thank you for your wisdom—from your mouth to my ears, "Never fear success, as it is often what gets in the way of following your true path." Gabby Karan DeFelice, we have been cooking, eating, and laughing for decades. My appreciation for you and our time together has no words. And Donna Karan, there is no other with a heart like yours; I honor and value the decades of edible conversation whether in your kitchen or at Urban Zen. Bridgette Butler, thank you for bleeding, sweating, crying, and laughing with me through graduate school—I couldn't have done it without you.

To every one of my clients and students over the years—I feel blessed to know all of you and to have had the opportunity to learn from all of your gifts. A teacher is always learning from her students. Thank you for inspiring me to be a better person and for encouraging me to speak up!

Peconic Public Broadcasting, WPPB 88.3 (and my sponsors), I am incredibly grateful that you all took a chance on me with *Stirring the Pot* radio. Amy Griggs

Kliger and Lee Ritchey, thank you for believing in me and helping shape my voice. Geir Magnusson, thanks for being my *Stirring the Pot* partner in crime. To my editor, Joanna Ng, and all the folks at Tarcher including Keely Platte, Sara Carder, and Brianna Yamashita *you* took a leap of faith and believed in this project when nobody else did; I am deeply grateful for and humbled by this incredible platform to share my message.

I may be the author, but it takes a village and I owe profound gratitude to many, including my dear friend and adored advisor Harriett Balkind, who always knows when to give me a swift kick in the ass; thank you for your unconditional love and support over every hill and valley. Barbara Close—you are not only my friend but also one of my greatest cheerleaders (without the pom-poms) and professional role models. To my lawyer, Jackie Eckhouse, I told you that someday I would write a book of my own—thank you for believing in me over the years, for all that you do and for knowing that Lauren Galit was the perfect fit. So to my literary agent LKG, it was a long arduous engagement, but worth it—I just love being "married" to you. Thank you for riding this roller coaster with me and keeping me buckled in along the way. I wouldn't want to take this journey with anyone else. James Blueweiss of Kismet Media Group, my manager and confidante, our collision in life was kismet—your support has been my missing ingredient in so many of my recipes. You truly brighten my days with laughter and cherished opportunity. Julie Negrin, our title brainstorm that summer eve in 2012 will never be forgotten; hopefully Martha in Iowa will read a book with this title. Brianne Halverson and Andy Shearer, I am so glad I know what I don't know—handing over the WTF bullhorn was a gift; so to my two amazing publicists, "you got me at hello." Jo Cooper (and A.N.), you sure know how to make a girl look good; thank you for my thoughtful and loving WTF web makeover (as well as your loving kindness).

To my writing muses—those food and nutrition junkies who loved me along the way, fed me information, reviewed my thoughts and words, and offered honest (and slightly painful) feedback to help shape the information in *What the Fork* making it as genuine as it could possibly be. I seriously could not have done this without any of you—your work is utterly commendable. Scott Cullen and GRACE Communications Foundation, words will never do my gratitude justice; you help make the food solution possible. Andrew Gunther (ten thousand times over) and the folks at Animal Welfare Approved (you know who you are), your insights and scrutiny of my every word were more helpful than I could have dreamed; thanks for steering me in the right direction for everything animal and beyond. My wonder twin, Sean Barrett of Dock to Dish, your passion for shining light in the deep waters of the sea has taken my knowledge to new levels—our shared journey is totally KFC. Marianne Cufone of Recirculating Farms Coalition, you are brilliant—I would like to live in your brain for a few days. Patty Lovera and the folks at Food and Water Watch—your understanding of the food system has helped me navigate something so complex. Dana Gunders of Natural Resources Defense Council, thank you for all that you do. Marc Jacobs, Lisa Lefferts and the folks at the Center for Science in the Public Interest, the team at the Environmental Working Group, Alexis Baden-Mayer of Organic Consumers Association and Mark Kastel of Cornucopia Institute—your expertise, insights and tools offered critical guidance. John Curry of Sweetener Solutions and Oregon State University's Kaci Buhl, thank you for giving the *dark side* a little sunlight—your constant availability to answer questions, review my words, and support my messaging was a gift. To the federal food regulating agencies, I can't count the number of times I called; thank you for your direct answers to my numerous inquiries. And to many other people who offered a few minutes here and there to answer my pressing questions, your time is appreciated. Lora Sporny, your encouragement over the years has given me permission to keep banging my drum. Mary Beth Augustine, our alliance and friendship is a true treasure—it's been fifteen years and you add constant insight and comedy to this edible journey. Kathie Swift, I am a devoted admirer and will always be blown away by your passion, knowledge, and wisdom—everyone should be so lucky to have a mentor like you; thank you for reading my words and being an integral part of my first book baby. Rebecca Katz (my dear Lucy), there is nothing like sharing this book pregnancy with you and giving birth at the same time; my every week has more yum (and belly laughs) because of you. John Bagnulo, wouldn't it be easier if we didn't care so much? But we do and your thoughtful input to this lettered canvas at the very beginning is greatly cherished. Marti Wolfson, recipe testing without you would have been a total nightmare! Your culinary intuition offered support and guidance through our grueling three days of food dancing. I am forever grateful. And Sarah Subrize, you are truly the answer to my prayers; thank you for your commitment to culinary nutrition and me. Always know that we will make it work and it will get easier.

To my friends who are part family—you have all seen me through so many ups and downs, have cheered me on along the way and offered outright TLC during the birth of this book. My "sister" Andrea Sanders, you have been my constant in life since the age of ten and I can assure you that I would never be where I am without you; you are treasured more than you will ever know. Tommy Grotta, you are the older brother I never had and the inspiration for my every day. Heather D'Agostino, our bond runs deep and my days would be empty without you—thank you for always being a moment away and enduring endless and sometimes pointless conversation. John D'Agostino, you are my number two—thank you for truly relishing in everything I cook and for washing the dishes. Kindra and Glenn Tatarsky, you may not be near but I feel you both every day and your encouragement over the years has helped me reach beyond my comfort zone. Shira Sacks Barzilay, simple and sweet—you are be.you.tiful says it all. Nancy Atlas, your many gifts add rhythm and color to my life.

Always know that wherever we go, it will be somewhere even if with a kid or two in tow. Elizabeth Yektai (my devoted recipe tester) and Sam Christie, thanks for your non-judgment, unwavering friendship, and always embracing my boys so writing and editing was a little bit easier. DJ Prager and Ann Marie Griffin, summers are extra special because of you—our endless feasts and family time is cherished. B. G. please know that your support over the years rests deep in my heart. Bruce Howard, thanks to my diva dog you are a constant in my life; your kindness is unprecedented and forever appreciated. Gen Kelsang Norden, thanks to you and Tara, I remain anchored through the nuances of life. And to all the other beautiful people who touch my heart, thank you for always checking in to see how I was weathering this sun shower—I felt you all cheering me on.

To my grandparents Seymour and Lorraine Schneidman, you made so many things possible in my life, including the gift of education that just can't be measured. To my brother, Ian, I loved cooking for you when we were kids (even if it was using my Betty Crocker oven) and I love cooking for you now. By the way, I will get you to eat that grape someday. Wendy, my rock-solid sister-in-law, thanks for always being there and for your devotion to dessert. Jaden, my little niece with a big personality, your unbreakable spirit through every farm stand, breakfast, and beverage bar is admirable; you are my Princess Anna. And to my nephews Isaac and Sawyer, thanks for always being our best customers.

Dad, thanks for always teaching me that there was no such thing as "I can't," that every problem had a solution and that I could do anything I set my heart to. You encouraged me to follow my dreams, no matter what they were. And Mom, you inspired creativity, always making the ordinary extraordinary. Thank you for regularly telling me that you seek without you the treasures you hold within—you helped me find my inner action hero. I am forever grateful to you both.

And to my husband, Rich Dec—it's no joke that out of tragedy comes beauty. Your courage has taught me more lessons than you know and your strength has given me strength. Thank you for always keeping my feet on the ground. I admire and love you so deeply. Charla really was a word—I just didn't know what it meant at the age of three. Jack and Hunter, my curious and courageous children, you inspire me each day to be the best mom I can be and to make a difference. May I pass this legacy on to you and may you both find purpose and happiness in this gift of life. And to my yellow labs and unconditional eaters, Blossom and the late Winnie, your company in the kitchen (and in life) centers my heart.

Notes

TOP-RATED TERMINATORS

1 "A Century of Ensuring Safe Foods and Cosmetics," http://www.fda.gov/AboutFDA/WhatWeDo/History/FOrgsHistory/CFSAN/ucm083863.htm (last updated April 2009).

2 "Generally Recognized as Safe (GRAS)," U.S. Food and Drug Administration, http://www.fda.gov/food/ingredientspackaginglabeling/gras/default.htm.

3 "CFR—Code of Federal Regulations Title 21," U.S. Food and Drug Administration, http://www.accessdata.fda.gov/scripts/cdrh/cfdocs/cfCFR/CFRSearch.cfm?fr=589.1001.

4 Bornehag, Carl-Gustaf. "Sources of Propylene Glycol and Glycol Ethers in Air at Home," *International Journal of Environmental Research and Public Health* 7 (12):4213–4237.

5 "Mission Statement—Center for Science in the Public Interest," Mission Statement—Center for Science in the Public Interest, https://www.cspinet.org/about/mission.html.

6 "USDA Fails to Verify Food Label Claims," Animal Welfare Institute, https://awionline.org/content/usda-fails-verify-food-label-claims.

CHEMICAL PRESERVATIVES

1 Hauter, Wenonah, and Mark Worth. *Zapped! Irradiation and the Death of Food* (Washington, D.C.: Food & Water Watch Press, 2008).

2 Bhaskaram, C. and Sadasivan G. "Effects of Feeding Irradiated Wheat to Malnourished Children." *American Journal of Clinical Nutrition*, no. 28: 130–135.

3 "Dr Pepper—Cherry Nutrition," http://www.drpepper.com/text/products/drpepper-cherry/nutrition/.

4 Mamur, Sevcan, Deniz Yüzbaşıoğlu, Fatma Ünal, et al. "Does potassium sorbate induce genotoxic or mutagenic effects in lymphocytes?" *Toxicology in Vitro 24* (3): 790–794.

5 U.S. Food and Drug Administration Code of Federal Regulations Title 21, http://www.accessdata.fda.gov/scripts/cdrh/cfdocs/cfcfr/cfrsearch.cfm?fr=130.9 (last updated June 1, 2013).

6 "Food, Nutrition, Physical Activity, and the Prevention of Cancer: a Global Perspective," the World Cancer Research Fund International, http://www.dietandcancerreport.org/cancer_resource_center/downloads/Second_Expert_Report_full.pdf.

7 "Chemical Cuisine," Center for Science in the Public Interest, http://www.cspinet.org/reports/chemcuisine.htm.

8 "Butylated Hydroxyanisole," U.S. Department of Health and Human Services, National
   Toxicology Program, http://ntp.niehs.nih.gov/ntp/roc/twelfth/profiles/butylatedhydroxy-
   anisole.pdf.
9 "Carcinogenesis Bioassay of Propyl Gallate," U.S. Department of Health and Human Services National Toxicology Program, Technical Report Series, 1982.
10 "Chemical Cuisine," Center for Science in the Public Interest.
11 "McDonald's USA Ingredients Listing for Popular Menu Items," McDonald's USA,
   http://nutrition.mcdonalds.com/getnutrition/ingredientslist.pdf (accessed May 2014).

ARTIFICIAL FLAVORS AND ENHANCERS

1 Reineccius, Gary. "What is the difference between artifical and natural flavors?" *Scientific
   American*, July 29, 2002.
2 U.S. Food and Drug Administration Code of Federal Regulations Title 21.
3 Schlosser, Eric. *Fast Food Nation: The Dark Side of the All-American Meal* (Boston:
   Houghton Mifflin, 2001).
4 Yamamoto, Kenji. "Novel Production Method for Plant Polyphenol from Livestock
   Excrement Using Subcritical Water Reaction," *International Journal of Chemical Engineering*, 2008, 1–5.
5 Pink Tentacle, "Ig Nobel Proze: Vanilla flavoring from cow dung," October 5, 2007,
   http://pinktentacle.com/2007/10/ig-nobel-prize-vanilla-flavoring-from-cow-dung/.
6 Mayo Clinic, April 2012, http://www.mayoclinic.org/healthy-living/nutrition-and-
   healthy-eating/expert-answers/monosodium-glutamate/faq-20058196.

ARTIFICIAL COLORS

1 U.S. Food and Drug Administration, http://www.fda.gov/ForIndustry/ColorAdditives/
   RegulatoryProcessHistoricalPerspectives/ (last updated December 17, 2009).
2 Ibid.
3 "CSPI Says Food Dyes Pose Rainbow of Risks—Newsroom—News from CSPI—Center
   for Science in the Public Interest," http://cspinet.org/new/201006291.html.
4 Kobylewski, Sarah, Ph.D., and Michael F. Jacobson, Ph.D. "Food Dyes: A Rainbow of
   Risks," 2010, Center for Science in the Public Interest, http://cspinet.org/new/pdf/food-
   dyes-rainbow-of-risks.pdf.
5 Schab, David, and Nhi-Ha T. Trinh. "Do Artificial Food Colors Promote Hyperactivity
   In Children With Hyperactive Syndromes? A Meta-Analysis of Double-Blind Placebo-
   Controlled Trials." *Journal of Developmental & Behavioral Pediatrics*, no. 25: 423–434.

ARTIFICIAL SWEETENERS

1 Nestle, Marion, PhD, MPH. *Safe Food: The Politics of Food Safety*. Updated and expanded
   ed. (Berkeley, CA: University of California Press, 2010).
2 Ibid.

3 "FAST FACTS Data and Statistics about Diabetes," American Diabetes Association, http://professional.diabetes.org/admin/UserFiles/0%20-%20Sean/FastFacts%20March% 202013.pdf.

4 Mayo Clinic, October 2012, http://www.mayoclinic.org/healthy-living/nutrition-and-healthy-eating/in-depth/artificial-sweeteners/art-20046936.

5 "The Pursuit of Sweet: A History of Saccharin," the Chemical Heritage Foundation, http://www.chemheritage.org/discover/media/magazine/articles/28-1-the-pursuit-of-sweet.aspx.

6 "About FDA: FDA History," U.S. Food and Drug Administration, http://www.fda.gov/AboutFDA/WhatWeDo/History/Origin/ucm055118.htm.

7 Arnold, D. L. "Two-Generation Saccharin Bioassays." *Environmental Health Perspectives, no.* 50:27.

8 Olney, John, Nuri B. Farber, Edward Spitznagel, et al. "Increasing Brain Tumor Rates: Is There a Link to Aspartame?" *Journal of Neuropathology and Experimental Neurology* 55 (11): 1115–1123.

9 Soffritti, Morando, Fiorella Belpoggi, Davide Degli Esposti, et al. "First Experimental Demonstration of the Mulitpotential Carcinogenic Effects of Aspartame Administered in the Feed to Sprague-Dawley Rats." *Environmental Health Perspectives* 114 (3): 379–385.

10 Soffritti, Morando, Fiorella Belpoggi, Davide Degli Esposti, et al. "Lifespan Exposure to Low Doses of Aspartame Beginning During Prenatal Life Increases Cancer Effects in Rats." *Environmental Health Perspectives* 115 (9): 1293–1297.

11 Bua, Luciano. "Aspartame administered in feed, beginning prenatally through life span, induces cancers of the liver and lung in male Swiss mice." *American Journal of Industrial Medicine* 53 (12): 1197–1206.

12 "Chemical Cuisine," Center for Science in the Public Interest.

13 "Chemical Cuisine, Asucelfame-K," Center for Science in the Public Interest, https://www.cspinet.org/reports/chemcuisine.htm#acesulfamek.

14 "Our Story," Splenda, http://www.splenda.com/story (last updated 2014).

15 "Sucralose Causes Cancer Concern," *Medical News Today*, http://www.medicalnews-today.com/articles/244603.php.

16 Strawbridge, Holly. "Artificial sweeteners; sugar-free but at what cost?" Harvard Health Publications, July 16, 2012, http://www.health.harvard.edu/blog/artificial-sweeteners-sugar-free-but-at-what-cost-201207165030.

17 Ibid.

18 http://www.neotame.com.

19 Kobylewski, Sarah, and Curtis D. Eckhert, PhD. "Toxicology of Rebaudioside A: A Review," PhD dissertation, University of California, Los Angeles, Department of Environmental Health Sciences and Molecular Toxicology, 2008.

SUGAR AND ITS MANY EUPHEMISMS

1 USDA National Organic Program Standards, http://www.ams.usda.gov/AMSv1.0/nop (last updated April 30, 2014).

2 "Roughly 180,000 deaths worldwide linked to sugary drink consumption." Harvard School of Public Health, http://www.hsph.harvard.edu/news/hsph-in-the-news/roughly-

180000-deaths-worldwide-linked-to-sugary-drink-consumption/ (accessed January 1, 2014); Qi, Qibin, Audrey Y. Chu, Jae H. Kang, et al. "Sugar-Sweetened Beverages and Genetic Risk of Obesity," *New England Journal of Medicine*, December 11, 2012; "Fact Sheet: Sugary Drink Supersizing and the Obesity Epidemic." Harvard School of Public Health, http://www.hsph.harvard.edu/nutritionsource/files/2012/10/sugary-drinks-and-obesity-fact-sheet-june-2012-the-nutrition-source.pdf.

3 Lustig, Robert H., Laura A. Schmidt, and Claire D. Brindis. "Public health: The Toxic Truth about Sugar." *Nature*, no. 482:27–29.

4 "What is GMO?" The NonGMO Project RSS, http://www.nongmoproject.org/learn-more/what-is-gmo/.

TRANS FATS (HYDROGENATED OILS)

1 Willett, Walter C., Meir J. Stampfer, JoAnn E. Manson, et al. "Intake of Trans Fatty Acids and Risk Of Coronary Heart Disease Among Women." *The Lancet*, no. 341:581–585.

2 "Dodd-Frank Wall Street Reform 324 in the last year." *Federal Register*, https://www.federalregister.gov/articles/2013/11/08/2013-26854/tentative-determination-regarding-partially-hydrogenated-oils-request-for-comments-and-for.

3 "FDA Targets Trans Fat in Processed Foods." U.S. Food and Drug Administration, http://www.fda.gov/forconsumers/consumerupdates/ucm372915.htm#pho.

4 "Rainforest Alliance." The and Palm Oil. http://www.rainforest-alliance.org/work/agriculture/palm-oil.

PESTICIDES

1 "Report confirms that U.S. food does not pose a safety concern based upon pesticide residues." U.S. Department of Agriculture, http://www.ams.usda.gov/AMSv1.0/getfile?dDocName=STELPRDC5049944.

2 "News Releases." Environmental Working Group, http://www.ewg.org/news/news-releases/2012/06/19/ewg-releases-2012-shopper%E2%80%99s-guide-pesticides-produce.

3 Reigart, J. Routt. "Book Review: *Pesticides in the Diets of Infants and Children* by a committee of the National Research Council," *New England Journal of Medicine*, no. 330:443–444.

4 "Executive Summary." Environmental Working Group, http://www.ewg.org/foodnews/summary.php.

5 Vandenberg, L. N., T. Colborn, T. B. Hayes, et al. "Hormones and Endocrine-Disrupting Chemicals: Low-Dose Effects and Nonmonotonic Dose Responses," *Endocrine Reviews*, December 6, 2012.

6 Smith-Spangler, Crystal. "Are Organic Foods Safer or Healthier Than Conventional Alternatives?: A Systematic Review," *Annals of Internal Medicine*, no. 157: 348–366. Brandt, Michelle. "Little evidence of health benefits from organic foods, Stanford study finds," Office of Communications & Public Affairs, http://med.stanford.edu/ism/2012/september/organic.html.

Notes 363

ANTIBIOTICS

1 "Animal Welfare." GRACE Communications Foundation, http://www.sustainabletable.org/274/animal-welfare.

2 "Superbugs Invade American Supermarkets," Environmental Working Group, http://www.ewg.org/meateatersguide/superbugs/?inlist=Y&utm_source=201306superbugs-subb&utm_medium=email&utm_content=first-link&utm_campaign=food.

3 "Record-High Antibiotic Sales for Meat and Poultry Production." Pew Charitable Trusts, http://www.pewhealth.org/reports-analysis/data-visualizations/record-high-antibiotic-sales-for-meat-and-poultry-production-85899449165.

4 "Animal Welfare." GRACE Communications Foundation.

5 "National Organic Program." U.S. Department of Agriculture, http://www.ams.usda.gov/AMSv1.0/ams.fetchTemplateData.do?template=TemplateC&leftNav=NationalOrganicProgram&page=NOPConsumers&description=Consumers.

6 "Superbugs Invade American Supermarkets," Environmental Working Group.

7 "Threat Report 2013." Centers for Disease Control and Prevention, http://www.cdc.gov/drugresistance/threat-report-2013/.

8 "About Animal Welfare Approved," Animal Welfare Approved About Comments, http://animalwelfareapproved.org/about/.

9 Andrew Gunther, conversation with author, November 2013.

HORMONES

1 Wolff, M. S. "Pubertal Assessment Method And Baseline Characteristics In A Mixed Longitudinal Study Of Girls." *Pediatrics* 126 (3): e583–e590.

2 "Steroid Hormone Implants Used for Growth in Food-Producing Animals," U.S. Food and Drug Administration, http://www.fda.gov/animalveterinary/safetyhealth/productsafetyinformation/ucm055436.htm.

3 Gunther, Andrew. "Would You Like Extra Ractopamine With Your Pork, Sir?" *Huffington Post*, December 5, 2012, http://www.huffingtonpost.com/andrew-gunther/would-you-like-extra-ract_b_2206643.html.

4 "Ractopamine: Human Health Effects," National Institutes of Health Toxicology Data Network (TOXNET), http://toxnet.nlm.nih.gov/cgi-bin/sis/search/a?dbs+hsdb:@term+@DOCNO+7441.

5 Stattin, P. "High Levels of Circulating Insulin-Like Growth Factor-I Increase Prostate Cancer Risk: A Prospective Study in a Population-Based Nonscreened Cohort." *Journal of Clinical Oncology* 22 (15): 3104–3112; Michaelsen, K. F. "High intakes of skimmed milk, but not meat, increase serum IGF-I and IGFBP-3 in eight-year-old boys." *European Journal of Clinical Nutrition*, no. 59:1211–1216; O'Neill, Bill. "In Methuselah's Mould." *PLOS Biology* 2 (1):e12.

6 "Hormones," GRACE Communications Foundation, http://www.sustainabletable.org/258/hormones.

7 "FishWatch," National Oceanic and Atmospheric Administration, http://www.fishwatch.gov/farmed_seafood/outside_the_us.htm.

8 Ibid.

9 Ibid.

10 Ibid.

11 "FishWatch." National Oceanic and Atmospheric Administration, http://www.fish-watch.gov/farmed_seafood/what_is_aquaculture.htm.

12 Food and Water Watch. "Antibiotics and Growth Hormones In Feed." Food Water Watch General, http://www.foodandwaterwatch.org/common-resources/fish/fishy-business/antibiotics-and-growth-hormones-in-feed/

GENETICALLY MODIFIED ORGANISMS (GMOS)

1 "Who We Are." Monsanto Company, http://www.monsanto.com/whoweare/pages/our-commitment-to-sustainable-agriculture.aspx.

2 "Food Wastage Footprint: Impacts on Natural Resources." The Food and Agriculture Organization of the United Nations (FAO), http://www.fao.org/docrep/018/i3347e/i3347e.pdf; "Think Eat Save," United Nations Environmental Program, http://www.thinkeatsave.org/index.php/about/about-the-campaign.

3 "Scientists Protest Unethical Clinical Trials of GM Golden Rice." Institute of Science in Society, http://www.i-sis.org.uk/SPUCTGM.php.

4 Tang G, Qin J, Dolnikowski GG, Russel RM, et al. "Golden Rice is an effective source of vitamin A," *American Journal of Clinical Nutrition*, no. 89:1776–83.

5 "Golden Rice Not So Golden for Tufts." *Science* magazine, http://news.sciencemag.org/asiapacific/2013/09/golden-rice-not-so-golden-tufts; "The Golden Rice Scandal Unfolds," Institute of Science in Society, http://www.i-sis.org.uk/goldenRiceScandal.php; "'Golden Rice' GM Vitamin-A Rice," Canadian Biotechnology Action Network, http://www.cban.ca/Resources/Topics/GE-Crops-and-Foods-Not-on-the-Market/Rice/Golden-Rice-GM-Vitamin-A-Rice.

6 "What is GMO?" The NonGMO Project RSS.

7 http://www.ers.usda.gov/data-products/adoption-of-genetically-engineered-crops-in-the-US#. VA4UGRdX6Z

8 http://online.wsj.com/articles/monsanto-under-attack-for-gmos-has-a-new-defender-1409777311

9 "Don Huber Interview—Roundup Ready GMOs—PATHOGEN NEW TO SCIENCE." https://www.youtube.com/watch?v=-nHCw36wIhs; "Is Monsanto Sowing the Seeds of Disease & Infertility? Scientist warns USDA of alarming rise in livestock infertility and crop diseases. Take action and tell the administration to halt the further planting of GMO crops!" Food Democracy Now, http://action.fooddemocracynow.org/sign/dr_hubers_warning/.

10 "Animal & Veterinary: Genetically Engineered Salmon," U.S. Food and Drug Administration, http://www.fda.gov/AnimalVeterinary/DevelopmentApprovalProcess/GeneticEngineering/GeneticallyEngineeredAnimals/ucm280853.htm.

11 "How'd we do that?" Okanagan Specialty Fruits Inc., http://www.arcticapples.com/arctic-apples-story/how-we-keep-apples-from-turning-brown.

FOOD LABELS 101

1 "Dodd-Frank Wall Steet Reform 324 in the last year." Federal Register, https://www.federalregister.gov/articles/2014/03/03/2014-04387/food-labeling-revision-of-the-nutrition-and-supplement-facts-labels.

2 Young, Dr. Lisa. "FDA proposes larger—more realistic—serving sizes for food labels." *The Portion Teller*, http://portionteller.com/fda-proposes-larger-more-realistic-serving-sizes-for-food-labels/.

3 Ibid.

4 "Guidance for Industry: A Food Labeling Guide (Ingredient Lists)," U.S. Food and Drug Administration, http://www.fda.gov/food/guidanceregulation/guidancedocumentsregulatoryinformation/labelingnutrition/ucm064880.htm#declare.

5 "Why Should We Eat Whole Foods?—An Article by Annemarie Colbin, Ph.D." http://www.foodandhealing.com/articles/article-wholefoods.htm .

6 "Melanie Warner: Where Do Vitamins Added To Processed Foods Come From? The Answer May Surprise You," https://www.youtube.com/watch?v=_Be2vwgPH-I.

7 "Farm Animal Welfare," American Humane Society, http://www.americanhumane.org/animals/programs/farm-animal-welfare.html; "Science-Based Standards," American Humane Association, http://humaneheartland.org/our-standards.

8 "Animal Welfare Standards for Dairy Cattle." file:///Users/stefanie/Downloads/Dairy%20Cattle-AHC%20Animal%20Welfare%20Standards_4_4_13r.pdf.

9 American Humane Association. "Animal Welfare Standards for Layers, Cage-Free, Aviary and Free-Range." http://humaneheartland.org/index.php?option=com_content&view=article&id=3&Itemid=106&jsmallfib=18dir=JSROOT/Animal+Welfare+Standards+-Full+Standards+%2B+Supplements

10 Ibid.

11 "Making History," Certified Angus Beef, http://www.certifiedangusbeef.com/brand/history.php (accessed May 2014).

12 "What Is Biodynamics?" Rethinking Agriculture, https://www.biodynamics.com/biodynamics.html.

13 United States Department of Agriculture: Agriculture Marketing Service, http://www.ams.usda.gov/AMSv1.0/ams.fetchTemplateData.do?template=TemplateC&leftNav=NationalOrganicProgram&page=NOPConsumers&description=Consumers.

14 "CNG—Brief History of Certified Naturally Grown," Certified Naturally Grown, http://www.naturallygrown.org/about-cng/brief-history-of-certified-naturally-grown.

15 United States Department of Agriculture: Agriculture Marketing Service.

16 "Food Alliance (FA)."—Food Alliance, http://foodalliance.org/.

17 United States Department of Agriculture: Agriculture Marketing Service.

18 "Gluten-Free Labeling of Foods." U.S. Food and Drug Administration, http://www.fda.gov/food/guidanceregulation/guidancedocumentsregulatoryinformation/allergens/ucm362510.htm.

19 "The Non-GMO Project Verified Seal." The NonGMO Project RSS, http://www.nongmoproject.org/learn-more/understanding-our-seal/.

20 United States Department of Agriculture: Agriculture Marketing Service.

21 Ibid.

22 Conversation and email exchange with American Grassfed Association, May 2014.

23 The Livestock Conservancy. http://www.livestockconservancy.org/index.php/heritage.

24 "Certified Humane—A Project of Humane Farm Animal Care." Certified Humane, http://certifiedhumane.org/.

25 "Food Irradiation: What You Need to Know," U.S. Food and Drug Association, http://www.fda.gov/Food/ResourcesForYou/Consumers/ucm261680.htm.

26 "What is Kosher?" Orthodox Union, http://oukosher.org/what-is-kosher-2/.

27 "USDA ERS—Report summary." U.S. Department of Agriculture, http://www.ers.usda.gov/publications/err-economic-research-report/err97/report-summary.aspx#.U3oodVhdWzs.

28 "What is the meaning of 'natural' on the label of food?" U.S. Food and Drug Administration, http://www.fda.gov/aboutfda/transparency/basics/ucm214868.htm.

29 Ibid.

30 Ibid.

31 "It's Official: An Action Alert," Organic Bytes #412, Organic Consumers Association, http://www.organicconsumers.org/bytes/ob412.html.

32 "Naturally Raised Marketing Claim Standards," U.S. Department of Agriculture, http://www.ams.usda.gov/AMSv1.0/ams.fetchTemplateData.do?template=TemplateN&rightNav1=NaturallyRaisedMarketingClaimStandards&topNav=&leftNav=GradingCertificationandVerfication&page=NaturallyRaisedMarketingClaims.

33 "Overview of Food Ingredients, Additives & Colors," U.S. Food and Drug Administration, http://www.fda.gov/food/ingredientspackaginglabeling/foodadditivesingredients/ucm094211.htm.

34 "Animal Byproducts Statement." Animal Welfare Approved, http://animalwelfare-approved.org/standards/animal-byproducts/.

35 "Meat and Poultry Labeling Terms," U.S. Department of Agriculture: Food Safety and Inspection Service (FSIS), http://www.fsis.usda.gov/wps/portal/fsis/topics/food-safety-education/get-answers/food-safety-fact-sheets/food-labeling/meat-and-poultry-labeling-terms/meat-and-poultry-labeling-terms.

36 Ibid.

37 "Nitrates and Nitrites: TEACH Chemical Exposure Summary," Environmental Protection Agency, http://www.epa.gov/teach/chem_summ/Nitrates_summary.pdf.

38 "National Organic Program," U.S. Department of Agriculture: Agricultural Marketing Service, http://www.ams.usda.gov/AMSv1.0/nop.

39 Ibid.

40 Ibid.

41 http://www.ams.usda.gov/AMSv1.0/ams.fetchTemplateData.do?template=TemplateC&leftNav=NationalOrganicProgram&page=NOPConsumers&description=Consumers.

42 "National Organic Program," U.S. Department of Agriculture: Agricultural Marketing Service.

43 "How Does Certified™ Compare to Fair Trade Certified™?" Rainforest Alliance, http://www.rainforest-alliance.org/agriculture/faq-fairtrade.

44 "Whole Grain Stamp," The Whole Grains Council, http://wholegrainscouncil.org/whole-grain-stamp.

45 "How to Spot Counterfeit Food," ABC News, January 12, 2013, http://www.abcnews.go.com/WNT/video/spot-counterfeit-food-18288837.

DO-IT-YOURSELF (DIY) PANTRY, FRIDGE, AND FREEZER REHAB

1 Mark Kastel, conversation with author, October 2013.

2 Nestle, Marion. *Food Politics: How the Food Industry Influences Nutrition and Health* (Berkeley: University of California Press, 2002).

3 Hauter, Wenonah. *Foodopoly: The Battle Over the Future of Food and Farming in America* (New York: New Press, 2012).

4 "The Dating Game: How Confusing Food Date Labels Lead to Food Waste in America," National Resources Defense Council, http://www.nrdc.org/food/files/dating-game-report.pdf.

5 Dana Gunders, conversation with author, October 2013.

6 "The Refrigerator Demystified," National Resources Defense Council, http://www.nrdc.org/food/files/dating-game-infographic.pdf.

SUPERMARKET STRATEGIES

1 "Understanding the Grocery Industry," U.S. Department of Treasury, http://www.cdfi-fund.gov/what_we_do/resources/Understanding%20Grocery%20Industry_for%20fund_102411.pdf.

2 "Front of Package Fail: labels tout healthier foods for kids, 84% studied flunk nutrition standards." Prevention Institute, http://www.preventioninstitute.org/focus-areas/supporting-healthy-food-a-activity/supporting-healthy-food-and-activity-environments-advocacy/get-involved-were-not-buying-it/735-were-not-buying-it-the-facts-on-junk-food-marketing-and-kids.html.

AISLE-BY-AISLE ACTIONABLES

1 "Bagged Salad: How clean?" *Consumer Reports*, March 2010, http://www.consumerreports.org/cro/magazine-archive/2010/march/recalls-and-safety-alerts/bagged-salad/index.htm.

2 "Mercury Levels in Fish," National Resources Defense Council, http://www.nrdc.org/health/effects/mercury/guide.asp.

3 "Organic Seafood: Fact or Fiction," Food Water Watch, http://www.foodandwaterwatch.org/common-resources/fish/seafood/labeling/organic-seafood-fact-or-fiction/.

4 "Endocrine Disruptors," National Institute of Environmental Health Sciences, http://www.niehs.nih.gov/health/topics/agents/endocrine/.

5 "News & Events: Bisphenol A (BPA): Use in Food Contact Application," U.S. Food and Drug Administration, http://www.fda.gov/newsevents/publichealthfocus/ucm064437.htm.

6 "Bottled Water," National Resources Defense Council, http://www.nrdc.org/water/drinking/qbw.asp.

7 "Why You Should Never Buy Disposable Water Bottles Again," Greatist, http://greatist.com/health/why-you-should-never-buy-disposable-water-bottles-again.

RECIPE REHAB

1 "Tip 6—Skip the non-stick to avoid the dangers of Teflon," Environmental Working Group, http://www.ewg.org/research/healthy-home-tips/tip-6-skip-non-stick-avoid-dangers-teflon.

2 Cliver, PhD, Dean O. "UC-Davis Food Safety Laboratory: Cutting Board Research," UC-Davis Food Safety Laboratory: Cutting Board Research, http://faculty.vetmed .ucdavis.edu/faculty/docliver/Research/cuttingboard.htm.

3 "To Nuke or Not? Microwave Facts," *Environmental Nutrition Newsletter,* April 2013.

4 "Importance of Healthy Breakfast: Why Skipping Is Harmful," WebMD, http://www .webmd.com/food-recipes/most-important-meal.

5 "The Juice on the Juicing Craze," *Environmental Nutrition Newsletter,* October 2012.

Index

Entries in *italics* refer to recipes.

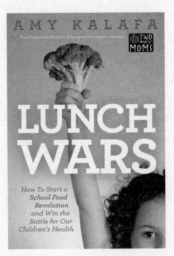